The Foaling PRIMER

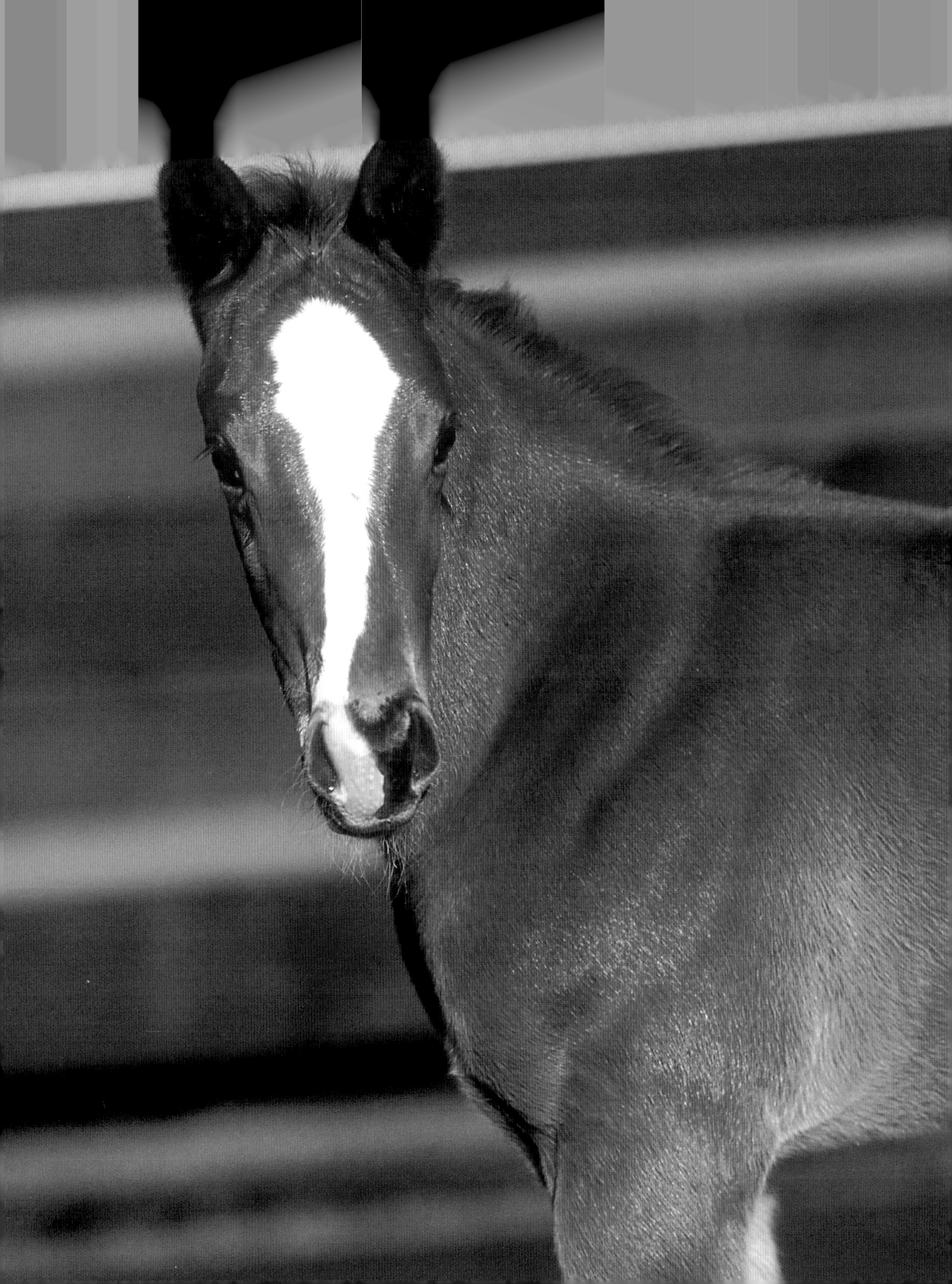

The Foaling PRIMER

A Month-by-Month Guide to Raising a Healthy Foal

Cynthia McFarland
Photography by Bob Langrish

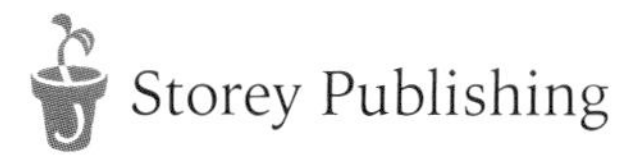

The mission of Storey Publishing is to serve our customers by publishing practical information that encourages personal independence in harmony with the environment.

Edited by Deborah Burns
Art direction and cover design by Kent Lew and Vicky Vaughn
Text design and production by Toelke Associates, Kristy MacWilliams, and Jennifer Jepson Smith
Illustrations by © Elayne Sears
Indexed by Jan Williams

Text copyright © 2005 by Cynthia McFarland
Cover and interior photographs copyright © Bob Langrish

All rights reserved. No part of this book may be reproduced without written permission from the publisher, except by a reviewer who may quote brief passages or reproduce illustrations in a review with appropriate credits; nor may any part of this book be reproduced, stored in a retrieval system, or transmitted in any form or by any means — electronic, mechanical, photocopying, recording, or other — without written permission from the publisher.

The information in this book is true and complete to the best of our knowledge. All recommendations are made without guarantee on the part of the author or Storey Publishing. The author and publisher disclaim any liability in connection with the use of this information. For additional information please contact Storey Publishing, 210 MASS MoCA Way, North Adams, MA 01247.

Storey books are available for special premium and promotional uses and for customized editions. For further information, please call 1-800-793-9396.

Printed in China by R.R. Donnelley
10 9 8 7 6 5 4 3 2 1

Library of Congress Cataloging-in-Publication Data

McFarland, Cynthia.
The foaling primer / by Cynthia McFarland ; photographs by Bob Langrish.
p. cm.
Includes index.
ISBN-13: 1-58017-608-8; ISBN-10: 1-58017-608-9 (pbk. : alk. paper)
ISBN-13: 1-58017-609-5; ISBN-10: 1-58017-609-7 (hardcover : alk. paper)
1. Horses—Parturition. 2. Veterinary obstetrics I. Title.

SF291.M385 2006
636.1'08982—dc22

2005021731

Dedication

To Jack, my companion and partner in all of life's adventures.

To my friends and family for your unfailing support, and to you, Mom, for introducing me to the magic of books so many years ago.

And to Sierra and Ben, the horses in my life, and my other four-legged "kids," a resounding thank-you for keeping me focused on what really matters.

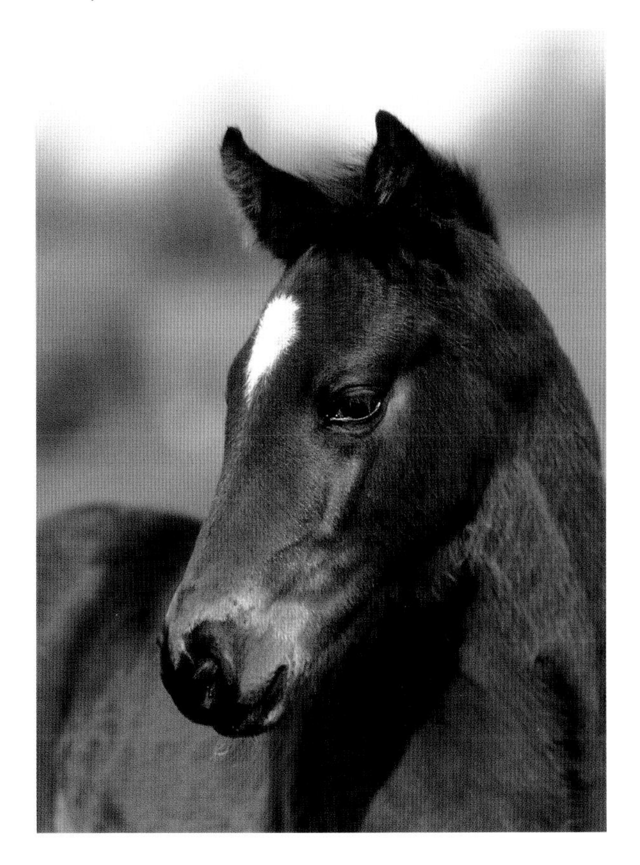

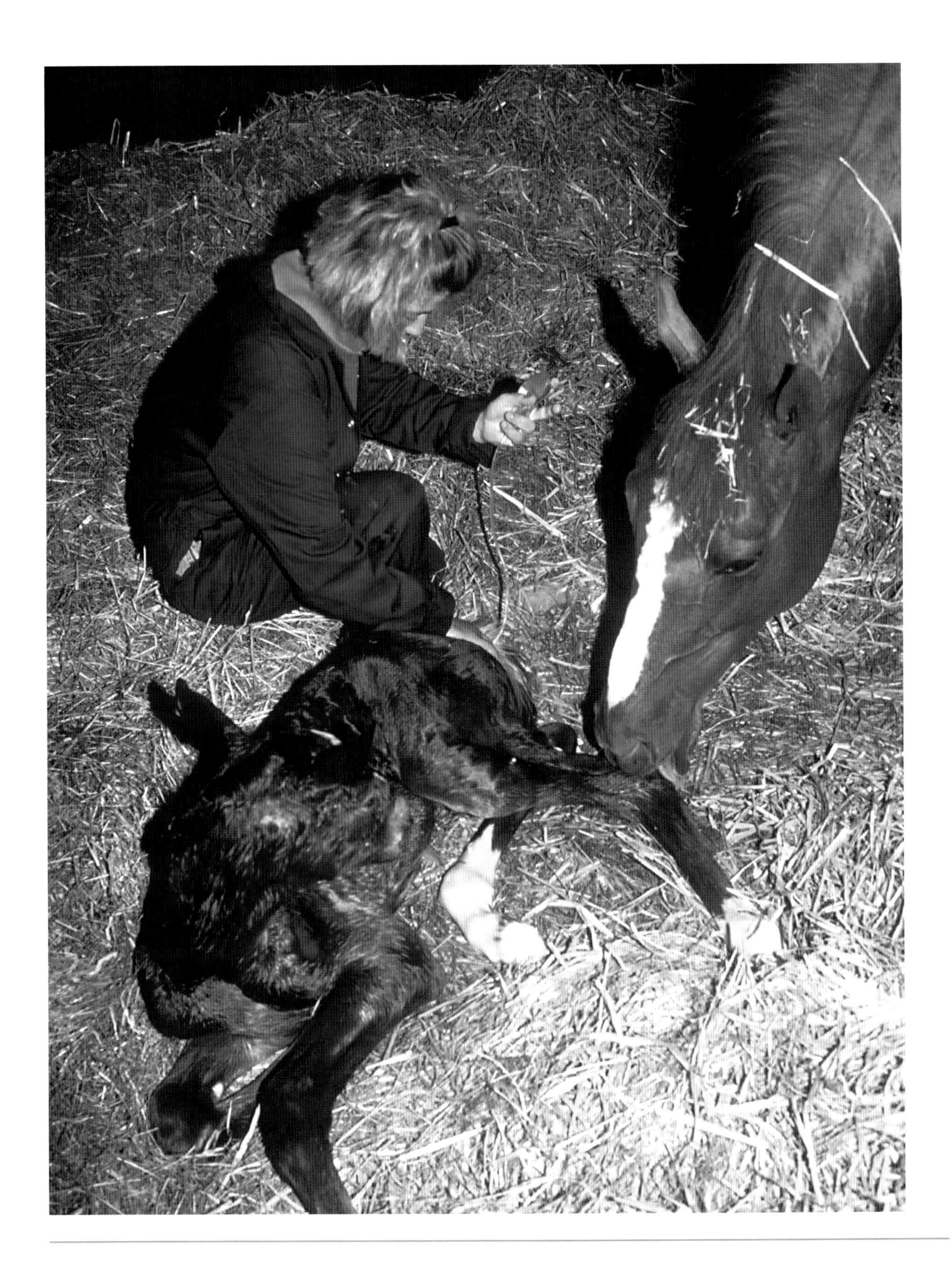

Contents

Foreword

I have been breeding and foaling mares for more than 50 years and naturally feel that along the way I have acquired a great deal of valuable information on the entire subject. Unfortunately, I can look back and remember making unintended mistakes that resulted in far too many losses and heartaches. If only someone had provided me with an opportunity to read a book such as this, no telling how much money I might have saved and how many disappointments with my foals I might have avoided.

"Horse folks" participating in the creation of the world's most beautiful animals all hope to be rewarded with magnificent, healthy foals. Nature or luck tries extremely hard to help us, but many of us absolutely abuse nature when we refuse to reinforce it with education. Unfortunately, our results are often sad and costly. On reading Cynthia McFarland's fascinating new book, illustrated with equally fascinating pictures, I am amazed at how cleverly she has documented all this important information on foals and made it so easy to digest. She has covered the many problems encountered by the novice and the expert from beginning to end, and has certainly reminded me of the vast amount of knowledge it takes to be successful, whether caring for one or many foals.

Cynthia shows complete understanding of all these problems through all stages of development, and every horse lover should be grateful for her desire to help them remember that each one of these chapters is equally important. The laws of nature are at all times respected and luck is always appreciated, but sometimes they both are absent. That's when we need to know exactly what is in this book.

Thank you, Cynthia, for giving both newcomers and old-timers a complete five-star read.

—Carol Harris
Bo-Bett Farm, Reddick, FL
Home of two-time AQHA SuperHorse Rugged Lark

Preface & Acknowledgments

This book is intended to serve as a helpful guide through the exciting and sometimes confusing process of gestation, foaling, and raising a foal. Use it as a handy reference and resource, and don't hesitate to ask questions of your veterinarian. There is no such thing as a dumb question.

As any horse owner quickly learns, there is not just one right way to do things. If you gather a dozen respected veterinarians, farm owners, and managers in one spot, you will hear a dozen variations on the same theme — and this doesn't mean any of them are wrong.

I have tried to write the guidebook I wish I'd had when I began the adventure of breeding, foaling, and raising foals. My hope is that it will give you direction, answer many of your questions, and prepare you for the rewarding experience of watching your foal enter the world and grow into a healthy young horse.

I am greatly indebted to those who graciously shared their expertise, offered their opinions, and generously gave of their time during my research. My heartfelt gratitude to Steven A. Murphy, DVM; Sharon J. Spier, DVM, PhD, Dipl. ACVIM, Associate Professor, Department of Medicine and Epidemiology, School of Veterinary Medicine, University of California at Davis; Kathleen Crandell, PhD, Kentucky Equine Research; Mark Shuffitt, University of Florida Cooperative Extension Service; Ken Breitenbecker; the American Association of Equine Practitioners; the American Quarter Horse Association; and the Appaloosa Horse Club. Thanks also to Mom, for your enthusiasm and thorough proofreading.

I truly appreciate the farm owners and horse owners who kindly allowed photographs of their horses to appear in this book: Bo-Bett Farm, BryLynn Farm, Lynn's Appaloosas, Horsefeathers Farm, Marablue Farm, Petty's Quarter Horses, Stanley White's Grandeur Arabians, Turtle Pond Farm, and Stonehedge Farm South. To Alexandria, Annette, Bobby, Casey, Caroline, Cindy, Dalton, Danielle, Evon, Lynn, Mary Jane, Nina, Shanea, and Dr. Murphy . . . you were perfect models!

— Cynthia McFarland

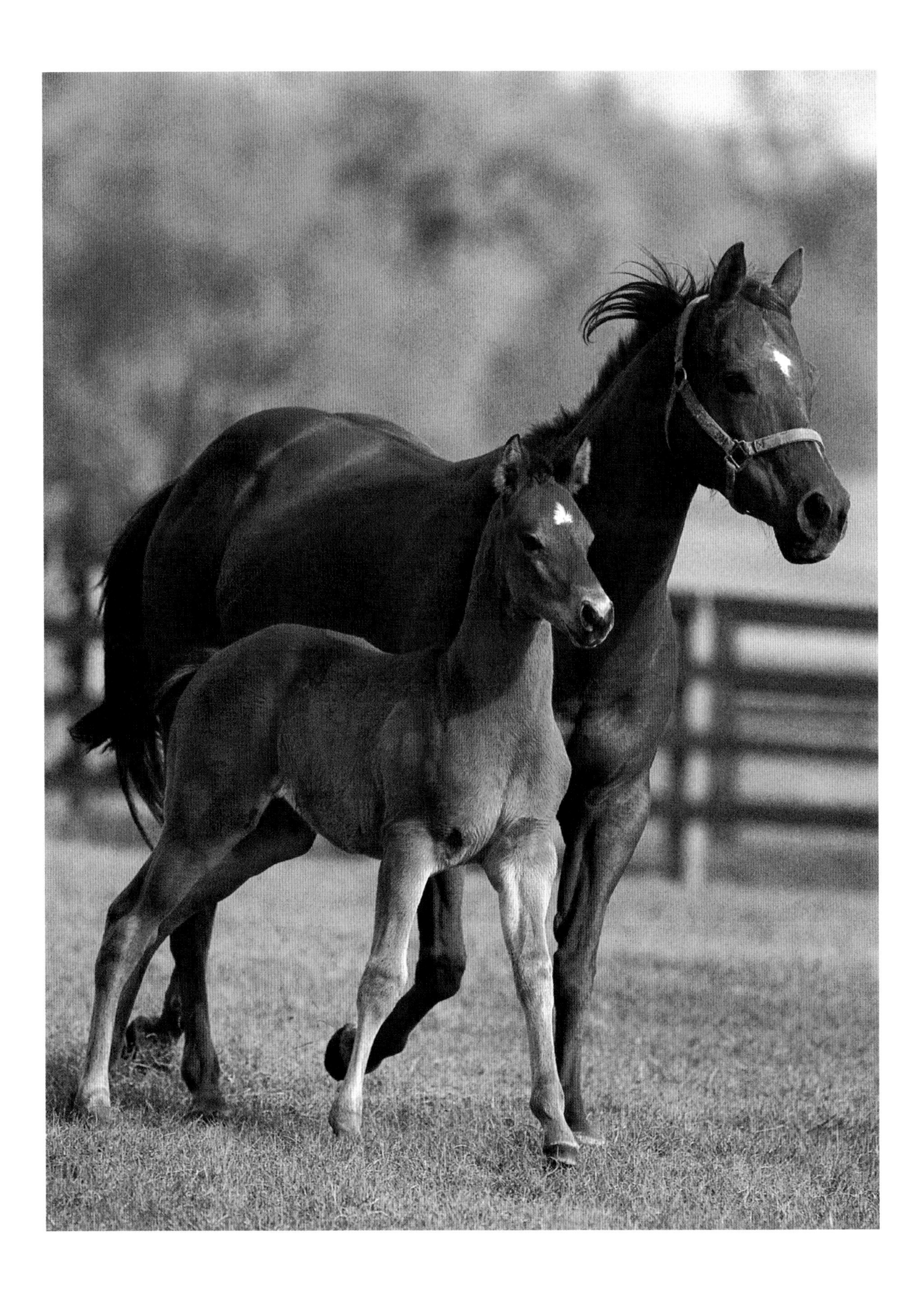

1

Getting Ready for the Big Day

It is springtime in horse country, and few sights stir the hearts of horse lovers more than that of mares and foals on good green pasture. It is an image filled with both the satisfaction of the moment and the promise of the future.

As the owner of a pregnant mare, you have put time and effort into choosing a stallion, breeding your mare, and caring for her over the months. Perhaps you bred your mare because she has such an outstanding pedigree that you want to carry on her bloodlines, or maybe you want to raise and train your own horse instead of buying one. It could be that you want to break into breeding and selling your own stock. For whatever reason, you now own a pregnant mare, and no doubt your mind is brimming with hopes and plans for the foal she is carrying.

If you show or participate in competitive events, you might be dreaming of raising tomorrow's champion. But you don't have to compete in a show ring to know the unique rewards in breeding and raising a beloved riding partner and companion. The journey from witnessing your foal's first wobbly steps to enjoying your friend and riding mount is one you will treasure for many, many years.

One thing is certain: You are sure to be counting down the days until the new foal's expected arrival. Because the average mare is pregnant for 343 days, your foal won't make his appearance until approximately 11 months and 11 days after the mare was bred. Welcome to the waiting game!

Will it be a colt or a filly? What color will he be? Will he have his dam's blaze and stockings or will he look more like his sire, with few white markings? Will she have her dam's kind, laid- back personality or be fiery, like her spirited sire?

Caring for the Pregnant Mare

Eleven months may seem like a long time to wait, but there is plenty you can do to fill the time. If you normally ride your mare, you can usually continue to take her on easy outings into the second trimester, unless your veterinarian says otherwise. Nonstrenuous exercise is beneficial to her, and throughout her pregnancy she should be turned out in order to exercise freely. Pregnancy and foaling will be

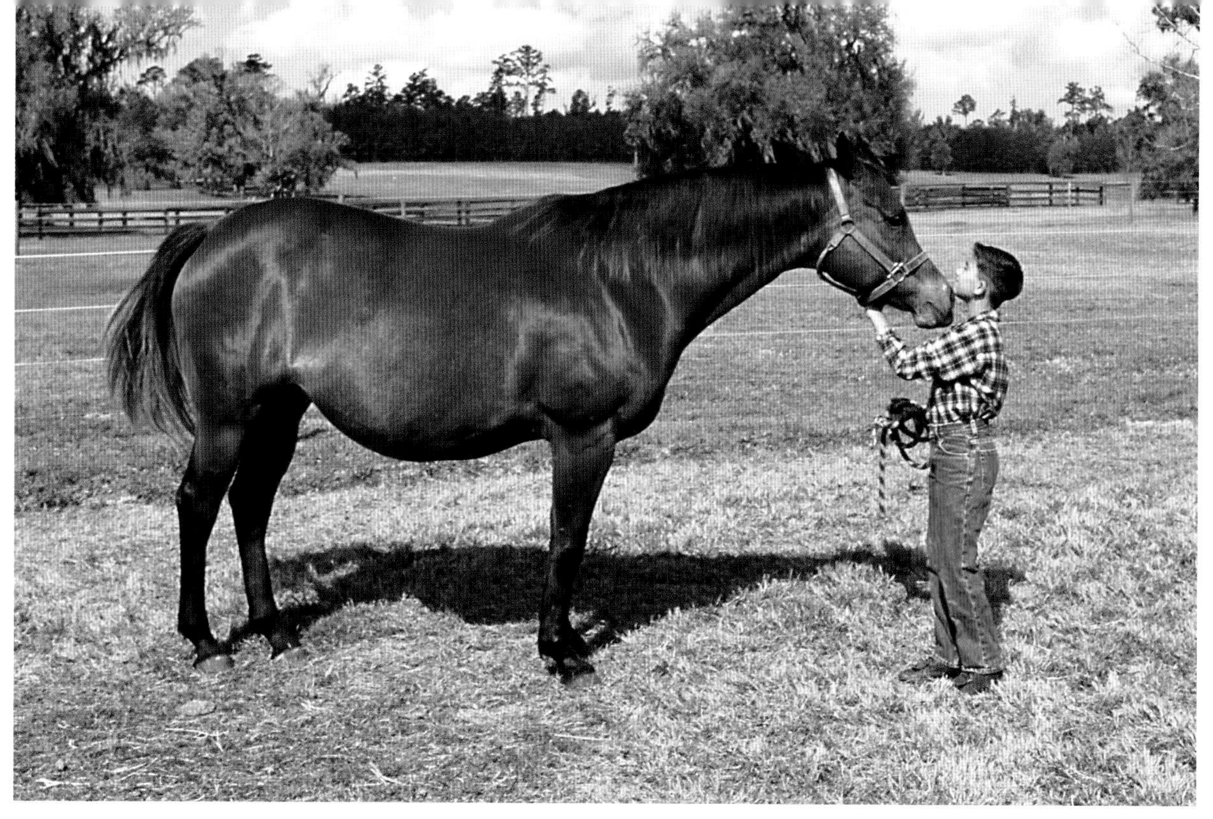

Although 343 days is the length of the average pregnancy, it's not uncommon for a mare to be "late."

easier if your mare is in shape and not overly fat or too thin.

Although she is "eating for two," you shouldn't have to change her feed ration during the first months of **gestation,** or pregnancy. During the first trimester, the average pregnant mare can be fed a maintenance ration. Her nutritional requirements will increase only slightly during the second trimester, as the fetus is not growing rapidly for these first eight months.

By the seventh month of gestation, the fetus is only about 17 percent of its birth weight. Sixty to 70 percent of the fetus's growth takes place during the third trimester, and in the last 2½ months of gestation, the fetus actually doubles in size. This is the most critical nutritional phase during pregnancy. For example, copper content in the mare's ration is essential during late gestation for healthy fetal bone development. If the mare doesn't receive adequate nutrients, she will deplete her own body stores.

The growing fetus builds up reserves of certain minerals such as copper, manganese, zinc, selenium, iodine, and iron during the last trimester. The foal will need these minerals during its first months of life. Because it is impossible to correct inadequacies by supplementing the mare and foal after birth, the mare must consume adequate amounts of trace minerals during her last months of pregnancy. Quality forage and a commercial balanced grain or concentrate ration designed for broodmares will contain the necessary nutrition during this important stage of gestation.

Purchase a weight tape at a feed or tack shop so you can determine your mare's approximate weight and can adjust her feed ration accordingly. Once the foal is born, the tape will also be helpful in measuring how the foal is growing.

Commercial feed labels give directions on how many pounds to feed according to your horse's size. As feed should always be fed by weight, not volume, it is advisable to purchase

BODY SCORING CHART: What Is Your Mare's Condition?

There are nine scores on the body-condition scoring system, with 1 being poor condition and 9 being extremely fat. Scoring is determined by looking at the horse from the side from a distance of about 15 feet. First look for noticeably visible ribs. If you don't see ribs, the horse's condition score is 5, which is considered moderate or better. (If the horse has a heavy coat, you will have to use your hands and not just your vision to check her condition.) A healthy pregnant mare should be a 6 or a 7 on the body scoring chart.

Some mares are easy keepers — that is, they gain and maintain weight easily; others are more difficult to keep weight on. If you have any questions about whether your mare is too fat or too thin while she is pregnant, don't hesitate to consult your vet.

Score 1: **Poor (abuse case)** — very prominent vertebrae, ribs, shoulders, withers, and tail head; extremely thin neck.

Score 2: **Very Thin (starved)** — prominent vertebrae and ribs; very thin neck, shoulders, withers, and tail head.

Score 3: **Thin (skinny)** — ribs readily visible; moderately thin neck, shoulders, and withers; prominent tail head.

Score 4: **Moderately Thin (underweight)** — light ridge along back; outline of ribs visible; neck, shoulders, withers moderately thin, some fat around tail head.

Score 5: **Moderate** — flat back (no crease or ridge); ribs easily palpable but not visible; shoulders and neck blend smoothly into body; rounded withers; moderate fat around tail head.

Score 6: **Moderately Fleshy (average)** — may have slight crease along back; ribs palpable but not visible; a little fat along withers, behind shoulders, and along neck; soft fat around tail head.

Score 7: **Fleshy (healthy)** — may have crease down back; ribs barely palpable; average fat along withers, shoulders, and neck; soft fat around tail head.

Score 8: **Fat** — crease down back; difficult to feel ribs; area around withers and behind shoulders filled with fat; noticeably thickened neck; fat along inner thighs; very soft fat around tail head.

Score 9: **Extremely Fat** (obese) — obvious crease down back; patchy fat over ribs; bulging fat along withers, behind shoulders, along neck, and around tail head.

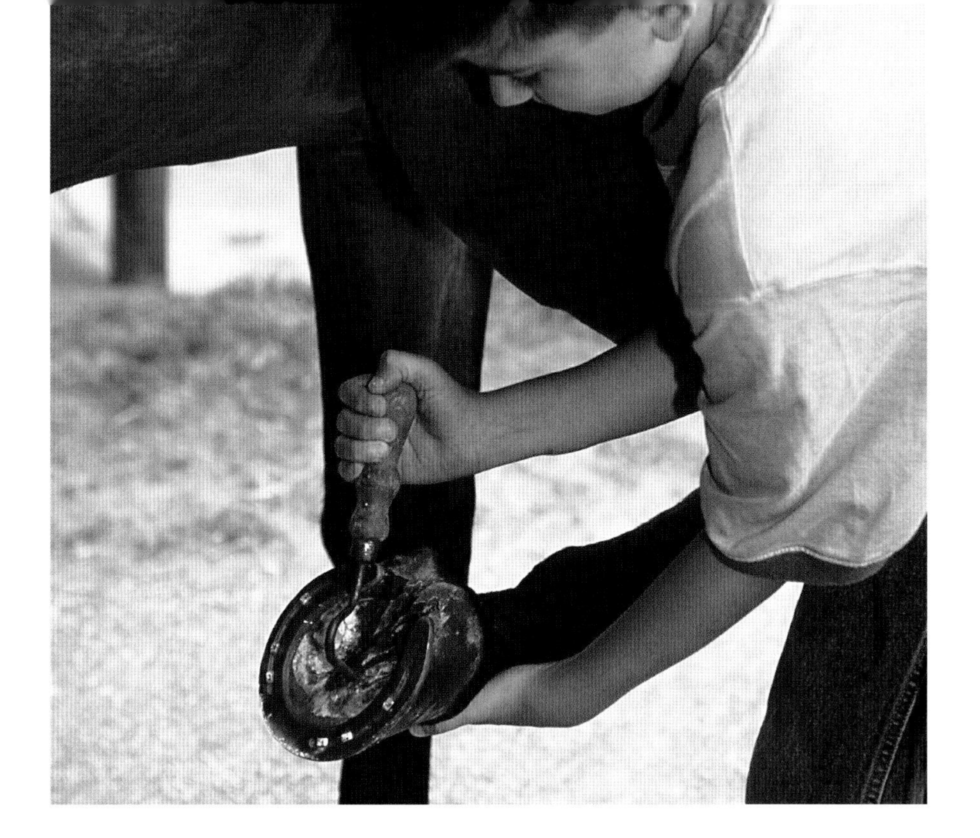

Keep up-to-date with your mare's hoof-care program.

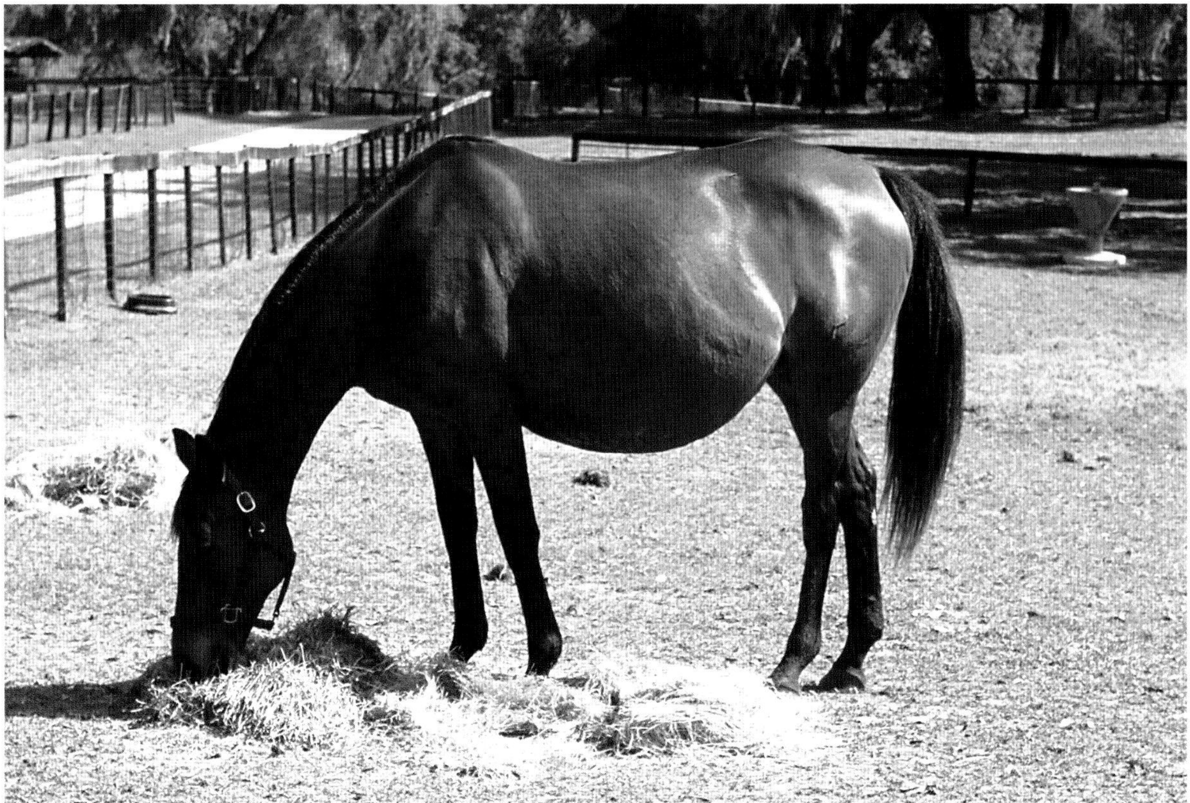

Although your mare is eating for two, you usually won't have to change her ration until the last trimester of pregnancy.

an inexpensive bathroom scale to keep in the barn. This makes it easy to weigh your feed ration and flakes of hay so you know exactly how much you are feeding.

Vaccinating the Pregnant Mare

A pregnant mare should be current on her vaccinations to protect her and her newborn foal. The veterinarian will tell you which vaccinations your mare should receive and when. For the greatest protection, vaccinate every spring and fall. Schedule her semiannual vaccinations for when she is five to six months pregnant.

To give your foal a healthy start, it's important to maximize the antibodies in the mare's

Watch Out for Fescue!

If your mare is grazing on a fescue pasture that is not endophyte-free, take her off this grass at least 90 days prior to foaling. Fescue grass often contains an endophyte fungus that causes serious complications during late pregnancy. These include abortion, thickened placenta, prolonged pregnancy, little or no milk production, and retained placenta after foaling.

Feeding the Pregnant Mare

Please note that all amounts given are approximate, as every mare is different. Rations should always be adjusted to meet your specific mare's needs.

The First 8 Months

Forage (hay and/or pasture): 1.5–2% of mare's body weight
Concentrate: 0–0.5% of mare's body weight
Total daily intake: 1.5–2% of mare's body weight
Example: (adjust to your specific mare's weight and needs)

- 1,000-pound mare x 1.5 to 2% of body weight in forage = 15 to 20 pounds forage (1.5 to 2 pounds forage per 100 pounds body weight)
- 1,000-pound mare x 0 to 0.5% of body weight in concentrate = 0 to 5 pounds concentrate (0 to 0.5 pounds concentrate per 100 pounds body weight)

Total feed ration: approx. 15–20 pounds/day

Last Trimester (months 9–11)

Forage: 1–1.5% of mare's body weight
Concentrate: 0.5–1% of mare's body weight*
Total daily intake: 1.5–2% of mare's body weight
Example: (adjust to your specific mare's weight and needs)

- 1,100-pound mare x 1 to 1.5% of body weight in forage = 11 to 16.5 pounds forage (1 to 1.5 pounds forage per 100 pounds body weight)
- 1,100-pound mare x 0.5 to 1% of body weight in concentrate = 5.5 to 11 pounds concentrate (0.5 to 1 pound concentrate per 100 pounds body weight)

Total feed ration: approx. 15–20 pounds/day

*Note that during these important last three months of gestation the amount of concentrate is usually increased in order to meet the mare's greater nutritional requirements.

colostrum (the first fluid produced by the mare, which is rich in protein and antibodies) by ensuring that she gets the booster shots the vet recommends four to six weeks before her foaling due date.

The vaccinations your mare requires will depend on where you live. Ask your vet about protection against the following diseases and when vaccinations are recommended.

Working with Your Vet

It's important to establish a good relationship with the vet **before** your foal is due, so she will become familiar with both you and your mare and won't be surprised in an emergency. Most important, she will already know how to find your mare!

- **Botulism** is caused by toxins produced by bacteria in soil and warm, moist conditions. Toxins may also be found in contaminated feed and water.
- **Eastern equine encephalomyelitis** (EEE, or sleeping sickness) is a viral disease spread by mosquitoes.
- **Influenza** (flu) is an upper respiratory disease caused by a virus.
- **Potomac horse fever** (PHF) is a potentially fatal disease caused by an organism that is thought to be ingested orally, possibly when a horse drinks from an infected pond or water puddle.
- **Rabies** is a fatal viral infection caused by a bite from or saliva contact with an infected animal. (Your vet may not want to give a rabies vaccine to a pregnant mare, so be sure to ask about this if you usually vaccinate for rabies.)
- **Rhinopneumonitis** (rhino) is caused by equine herpes virus and can cause abortion, respiratory disease, and disorders of the nervous system. Brood mares should be vaccinated at 5, 7, and 9 months of gestation.
- **Rotavirus A** causes diarrhea in foals. Mares should be vaccinated at 8, 9, and 10 months of gestation.
- **Strangles** is a bacterial respiratory disease. Ask your vet about vaccinating, especially if you have a young mare and/or live where strangles is endemic.
- **Tetanus** (lockjaw) is caused by bacteria. Infection can occur when a wound is contaminated.
- **West Nile virus** is a potentially deadly disease spread by mosquitoes. Depending on where you live, your vet may recommend West Nile boosters more than twice a year.
- **Western equine encephalomyelitis** (WEE, or sleeping sickness) is a viral disease spread by mosquitoes.

Deworming the Pregnant Mare

Your mare must still be protected from internal parasites during gestation, but be sure you use a deworming product that is labeled safe for pregnant mares.

Depending on your geographic area and the number of horses in your mare's environment, deworm her every four to eight weeks. It's important to rotate among categories of deworming products; if you use only one product, parasites may become resistant. When you read the label, you'll see that not all products eliminate the same parasites. Because tapeworms can cause serious problems, twice a year use a dewormer specifically designed to kill these worms. Your veterinarian can give you advice on which dewormers to choose, along with when and how often to use them. For the pregnant mare, a vet will most likely tell you to rotate between avermectin and pyrantel dewormers. Thirty days from the mare's due date, deworm her with a product that is safe for mares in the last trimester. Then deworm her once more on the day the foal is born with an avermectin class dewormer, such as ivermectin.

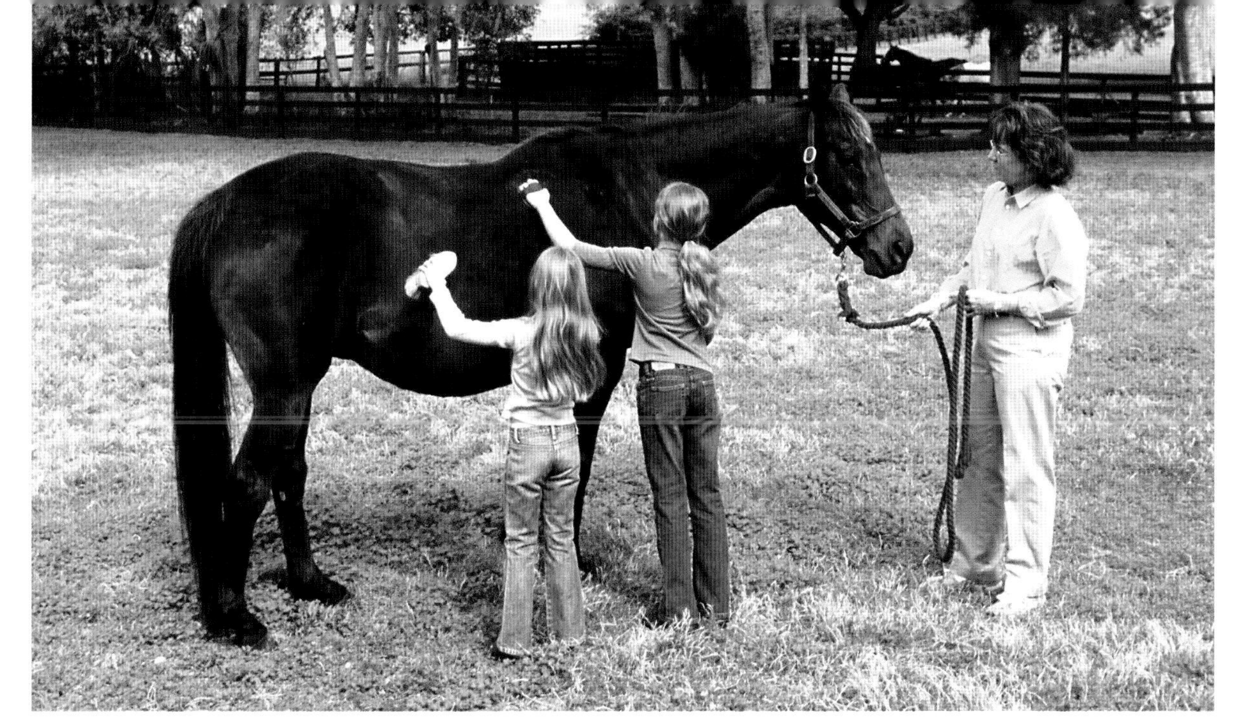

Your mare will appreciate being groomed and cared for while she is pregnant.

Preparing the Foaling Area

With time winding down until the big day, you'll want to make sure you have everything prepared before the foal arrives, beginning with the foaling area.

In the wild, a mare leaves the herd and finds a secluded place for the birth of her foal. She will look for a place where she feels safe and secure. Because most domesticated horses are confined and cannot choose where they want to foal, it's up to you to provide a comfortable place that is quiet, clean, and safe. For example, if there are dogs around the barn, keep them out of the area as the mare approaches foaling time.

Whether you keep your mare at home or board her out, you will need to plan ahead for a proper foaling area, in which the mare will take up residence no less than four weeks in advance of foaling. This time period will allow her body to produce the antibodies in her colostrum that will provide the foal with

Caslicks Procedure

A **Caslicks** is a common veterinary procedure that prevents infection and is performed on pregnant mares under local anesthetic. It involves cutting away a thin piece of tissue on the edges of the vulva and suturing the edges together, leaving an opening large enough for urination. If your vet determines that the mare should have a Caslicks, it will be performed after she has been checked "in foal."

A Caslicks should be opened about 30 days from the mare's due date — earlier if you notice her udder is beginning to fill out. It is very important that the vet cut open the Caslicks *before* the foaling; otherwise, the mare may severely injure herself and the baby during delivery.

immunity to possible disease-causing organisms present in the foaling environment.

Even if your mare is kept with other horses while she is pregnant, you should create a separate area for foaling, both for her safety and for that of her newborn. Mares and geldings have been known to injure and even kill foals, so you will want your mare and her newborn to be protected in their own pen or paddock. A double fence between pastures or pens is ideal, so other horses can't reach over the fence into the foaling area. A mare may injure her own foal just by aggressively defending him from other horses. When the foal is a little older, the pair can be turned out with other mares and babies.

Foaling Outdoors

At most large breeding farms, mares deliver their foals inside a barn, but there is nothing wrong with nature's way of foaling outdoors, provided the weather is mild and dry and that it takes place in an area that meets certain requirements.

It must have strong, safe fencing to protect the mare and foal from anything that could harm the vulnerable new foal, such as other horses, dogs, or roaming animals. The safest fencing for young foals is diamond-V mesh. Because the openings are small and V-shaped, they are too small for even little foal legs to get caught in. "Nonclimb" wire fencing is also popular, but the openings are two inches by four, which is not as small as the diamond-V mesh.

It is better to avoid standard field fencing — the holes are too large, making it easy for a horse to poke a leg through. Metal pipe or plain board fencing is often used on farms, but neither is a wise choice for the foaling area because a foal may be able to slip under or through, and if the mare lies down next to the fence, she or the foal can become caught. In addition, this type of fencing will not keep out

All-Important Colostrum

Foals have no defenses against bacteria and viruses when they are born, which is why it is critical that they receive colostrum. Unlike a human baby, who is born into a fairly sterile environment, a foal immediately comes into contact with germs and bacteria. Colostrum provides protection as the foal's small intestine absorbs the antibodies it contains within the first 24 hours of life. After the first day, the foal's gut can no longer process these antibodies, so make sure he receives colostrum shortly after birth.

Some mares "leak milk" for several days before foaling and lose some of this valuable colostrum. Talk to your veterinarian if you are concerned about this possibility. Many large farms collect colostrum from foaling mares and freeze it for use in just such a situation. Colostrum will maintain its value for up to two years if it is properly frozen. (See chapter 4 for more information on frozen colostrum for use in bottle-feeding.)

Colostrum supplements are available at your feed store, but you should understand that these do not fully replace real colostrum from a mare. These products vary in quality, so ask your veterinarian for recommendations if a supplement is needed.

other animals that might try to harm the newborn.

Barbed- or smooth-wire fencing should never be used around foals or young horses, especially in a small area. Some large ranches do use barbed-wire fences, but this is usually in pastures that cover many acres, so the horses are rarely in close proximity to the fence. To be on the safe side, rule out barbed-wire fencing when it comes to horses.

Electric fencing is also not suitable for the foaling area. You should use electric fencing only with adult horses that are familiar with and respect this type of fencing.

An outdoor foaling area ideally should be grass, not dirt. Keep other horses out of this area for at least several weeks before foaling to decrease the chances of contamination.

Most mares end up foaling at night, so if you use an outdoor area, make sure it is well lit. The space should be small enough that the lights illuminate the entire area (but not so intense as to deter the mare from entering her first stage of labor).

Foaling Indoors

If you decide to foal your mare inside, you'll need to prepare the stall well ahead of time. When he is born, the only protection the foal has against disease comes from his mother's colostrum. Bacteria can be ingested or inhaled, or it can enter the foal's body through his navel stump if it is not properly treated; thus, it is critical that your stall or foaling area be as clean as possible.

Proper Cleaning and Disinfecting

If the stall walls are wood, cleaning is much more difficult because wood is porous. To create a nonporous surface, paint the wood with two coats of marine-quality varnish or a similar sealant, following the manufacturer's directions. Painting concrete block walls with enamel paint will make them even easier to clean and disinfect.

To clean the foaling stall, first muck out all of the bedding. Remove any buckets, feed tubs, and other equipment. Then scrub all surfaces using water and detergent, working from the top of the walls to the floor. Rinse thoroughly, then repeat if there is any dirt or manure still visible.

Once you have cleaned the walls and floor with detergent and water, let the stall dry. Fans help speed up the drying process.

After the stall is dry, follow directions on the label and spray all surfaces with a disinfectant such as One Stroke Environ or Tek-trol; both have proved effective in horse barns. (These disinfectants are available through chemical supply stores, veterinary supply distributors, and some feed and supply stores.) Again, allow the stall to dry completely. If floors are dirt, spread barn lime on any moist areas. It is best if the stall can remain empty — unused and without bedding — for a week or so before your mare uses it for foaling.

Some farms use padded rubber cushions attached to the walls in case the mare or foal bumps against them, and these also need to be thoroughly cleaned and disinfected.

You want the stall to be "foal-proof." Remove anything that has the potential to be dangerous to the foal. Look for broken or splintered pieces of wood, nails, sharp hooks, brackets for buckets or feeders, screw eyes, salt-block holders, and pieces of metal. It helps if you actually get down on your hands and knees to take a look around at the level of the foal when he's lying down, rolling, or trying to stand up.

Bedding

Straw or bedding hay is best for a warm, soft foaling bed. Whichever bedding you choose, make sure it is not moldy or dusty. Straw should be bright and long-stemmed. Good choices are high-quality wheat and rye straw.

Although shavings are popular as horse bedding, do not use them in the foaling stall, as they will stick to the wet newborn and possibly interfere with his respiration. Don't use sawdust, either; it is dusty and has even smaller potentially irritating particles.

If you normally use shavings for bedding, switch to straw or bedding hay for the foaling phase. You can use shavings after the foal is a few days old. Be sure to buy shavings with as little dust as possible. And keep an eye on the new baby: some foals will eat shavings, which can lead to colic, stomach upset, or impaction. Wood harbors bacteria and contains resins that can cause skin allergies. Some horses are more sensitive to irritants than others. If you use shavings and your mare or foal develops bumps or hives, switch to another type of bedding immediately.

If your mare will be foaling in winter and you live in a cold climate, you may need to use a heat lamp for added warmth. Use infrared heat lamps in place of the regular socket light bulbs. *It is of utmost importance that you place the heat lamps away from anything flammable, such as bedding or hay.*

If you need more than one source of illumination and an extension cord is required, be very careful that the cord is out of reach of both mare and foal *at all times.* Make sure the barn is fully equipped with smoke detectors and fire extinguishers.

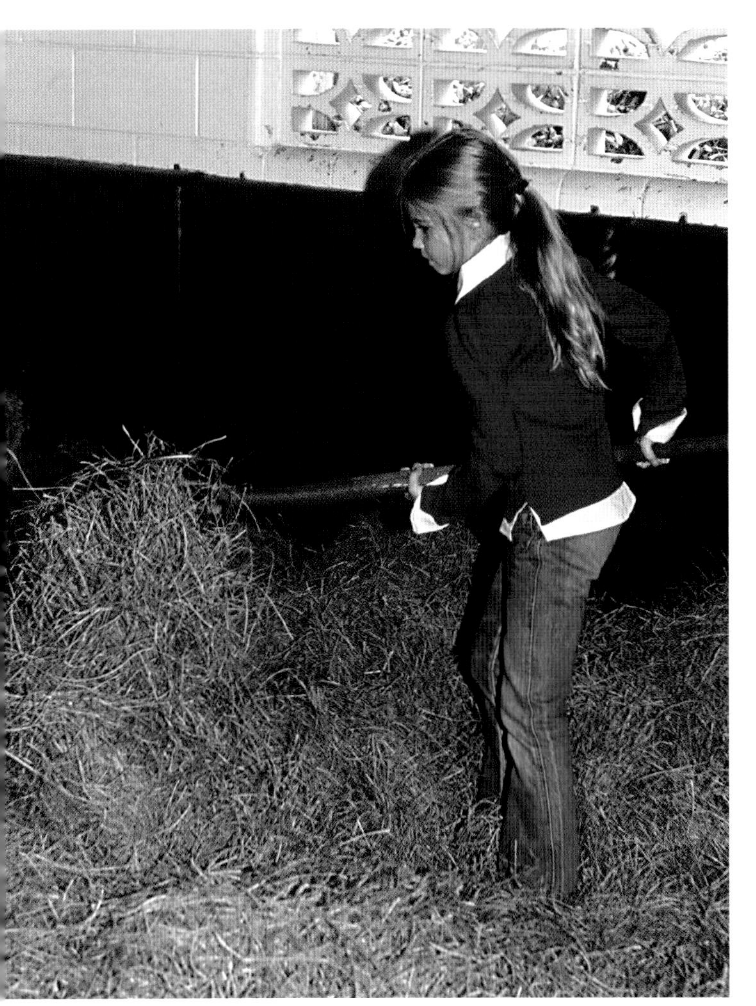

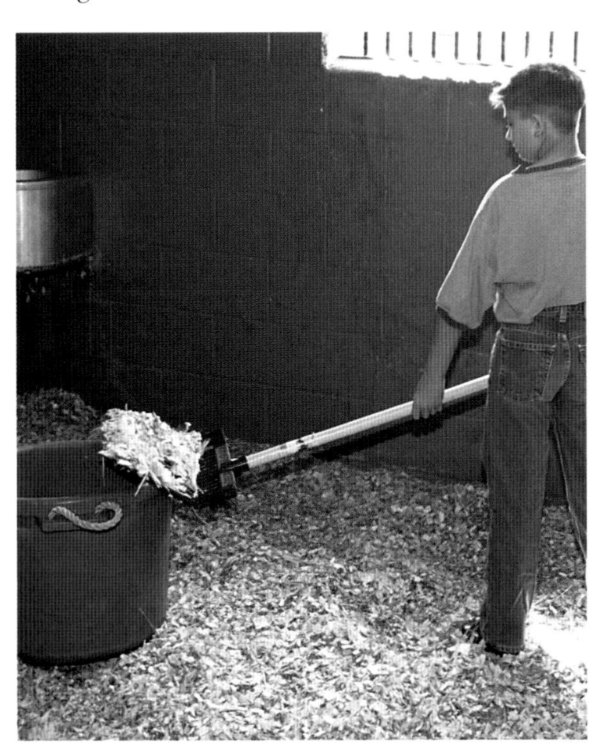

Don't use shavings for foaling. They are fine, however, when the foal is a few days old.

Straw or bedding hay is the best choice for the foaling stall.

Final Days before Foaling

If you pay attention, your mare will give you definite signs of the impending birth in the final days before she foals. Each mare reacts individually, but the following changes usually occur seven to ten days prior to the due date.

- The mare's udder will fill out and become more dense.
- The muscles over her croup and tail head will soften and relax (become "Jell-O-like").
- A quiet mare may become more active or restless; an energetic mare may seem quieter.
- The mare will pass a small amount of dense white or off-white mucus. This mucus plug is typically passed within 72 hours of foaling.

A significant amount of discharge is not normal. If you see this, tell your vet. You should also call the vet if there is any reddish discharge late in the pregnancy, as this is not normal and could signal a problem.

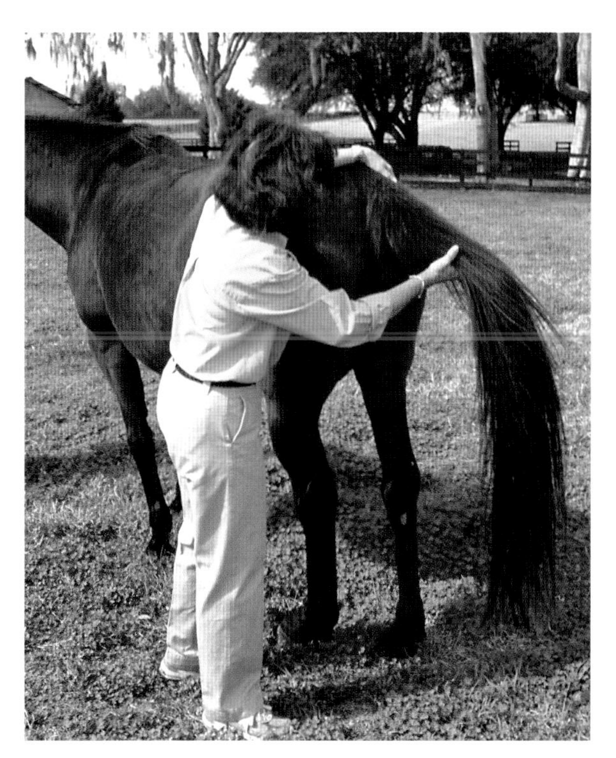

The muscles over the mare's croup and tail head relax and loosen as she gets closer to foaling.

Cleaning the Udder

About a week before the due date, use a sponge and gently wash the mare's udder with warm water and a mild soap, such as Ivory. You aren't disinfecting, but rather performing a basic cleanup. Don't wait until just before your mare is ready to foal and has a big, tight udder. She'll be uncomfortable at that stage and won't appreciate your attentions. Also, you don't want to remove all of the mare's natural scent from her udder — this odor helps the foal find his "target" when he nurses for the first time.

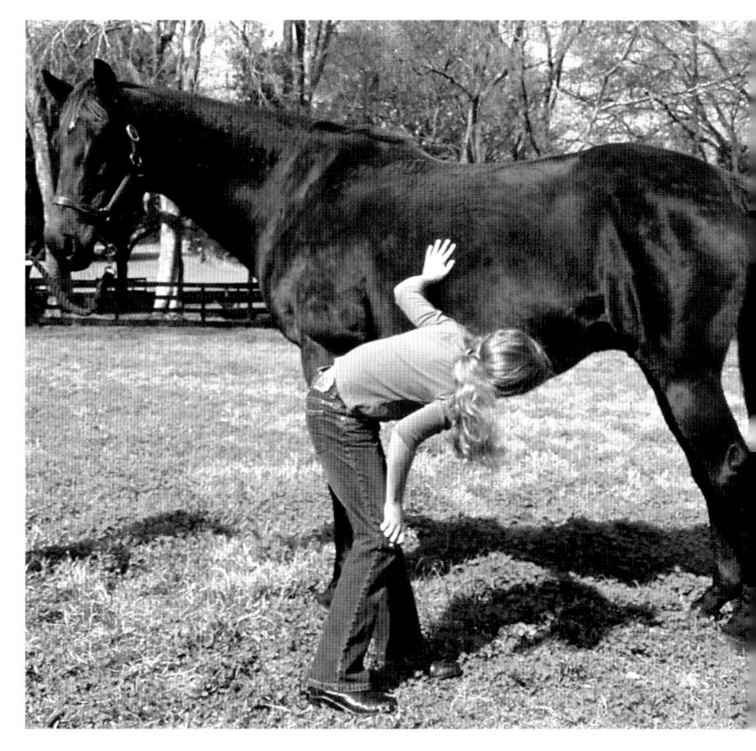

In the days before she foals, the mare's udder will fill out as she starts making milk.

Have Emergency Numbers Handy

Keep a list of numbers ready by the phone so you don't need to look for one if you are in a hurry. Include the emergency number of your regular veterinarian, as well as that of a second, backup vet. If there is an equine hospital or a vet school hospital nearby, it is a good idea to have this number handy, too. You should also list the phone number of a reliable van company or have access to a truck and horse trailer should the rare situation arise that the mare must be shipped to a veterinary hospital.

Preparing Your Supplies

Have ready everything you need for foaling before the due date. You can keep your supplies in a cupboard during the year, but as the birth day nears, stock them in a portable and convenient grooming box or a plastic toolbox.

Foaling Alarm Systems

The last thing you want is to miss the arrival of your foal. To ensure that you are present for the big moment, consider a foaling alarm system. There are several systems on the market, with different methods of operation. Most employ a transmitter and receiver to sound an alarm or to call a phone number you program into the system. If you decide to use an alarm system, ask your vet to make a recommendation. (See the appendix for more information.)

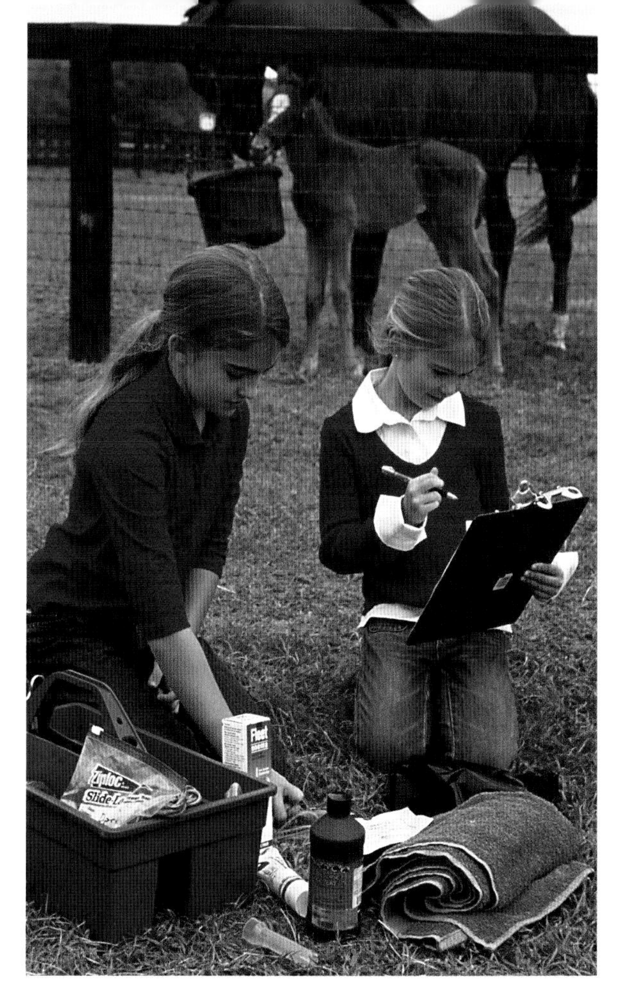

Assemble your foaling supplies ahead of time so you'll be ready for the big moment.

If Your Mare Is Overdue

Although the typical equine pregnancy lasts a little more than 11 months, or 343 days, mares have foaled as early as 300 days and as late as 380 days without serious problems. As a rule, though, the more your mare deviates from the standard 343 days, the greater the chance of something going wrong. If your mare is a week past her due date, the vet will probably want to perform a rectal exam to check the position of the foal and confirm that everything is progressing normally.

There are several brands of testing kits designed to predict when a mare will foal. These kits require just a few drops of milk in order to test the calcium level and include easy-to-follow instructions. Such tests are *usually, but not always,* accurate to within 24 hours. There's nothing wrong with using such a test and it can sometimes give you a heads-up, but *don't rely on this test alone!* Some mare owners have performed the test, left the mare alone, and returned after a few hours only to find that the baby has already arrived.

Approximate Length of Gestation

Mouse — 21 days
Rabbit — 31 days
Gray squirrel — 44 days
Cat — 60 days
Dog — 63 days
Sheep — 148 days
Black bear — 210 days
Woman — 280 days
Cow — 285 days
Mare — 343 days
Sperm whale — 480 days
Elephant — 680 days

Checklist of Foaling Supplies

- ☐ Terry cloth bath towels or half-size bath towels.
- ☐ Stainless-steel bucket.
- ☐ Liquid detergent such as Ivory, Dawn, or Joy.
- ☐ Roll of cotton.
- ☐ Baling twine or strong string.
- ☐ Scissors.
- ☐ Enemas (any enema safe for children is fine; a phosphate enema is best).
- ☐ Tincture of Iodine* or Nolvasan (chlorhexidine solution) for dipping navel. If you use iodine, be sure to have a new, unopened bottle. Always dispose of any bottles of leftover iodine each year.
- ☐ Small plastic containers or 60 cc plastic syringe cases (for dipping foal's navel). Putting iodine in the container will enable you to dip and thoroughly saturate the navel stump. You need to dip the stump into the iodine, not just swab or spray iodine on it!
- ☐ Umbilical clamps or rubber bands (if a foal's navel bleeds abnormally).
- ☐ Digital thermometer.
- ☐ Obstetrical sleeves or plastic rectal sleeves.
- ☐ Disposable tail wrap or gauze bandage (for wrapping tail).
- ☐ Disposable latex gloves.
- ☐ Obstetric lubricant or K-Y Jelly.
- ☐ Small blanket or old down vest (in case you have to keep the foal warm on a cold night).
- ☐ Flashlights and fresh batteries (in case of power failure).
- ☐ Cell phone or cordless phone, fully charged.
- ☐ Phone numbers of vets, experienced foaling person, equine hospital (keep list next to the phone).

*Some vets use 2 percent iodine; others swear by the stronger 7 percent. If you decide to dip the navel in iodine, ask your vet to recommend the strength.

Foal-ALERT, shown here attached to the mare, is one foaling system that will sound an audible alarm or dial a programmed number to let you know when foaling starts.

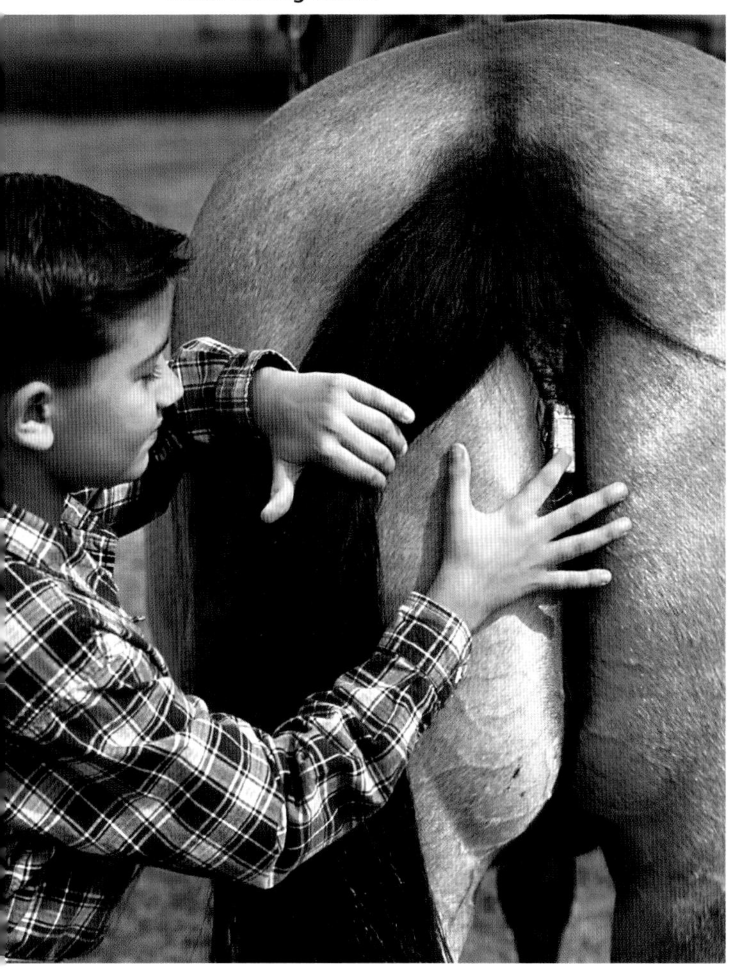

Countdown to Foaling

2 to 3 weeks after breeding

- Schedule a veterinary ultrasound exam to determine if your mare is pregnant. If the ultrasound shows the presence of twins, the vet will usually "pinch" one, as multiple births are not encouraged in horses. At this exam, the vet will tell you when the mare should be checked again. More than one pregnancy check is strongly recommended; it is not uncommon for mares to lose a pregnancy in the very early stages. If this happens and you discover it soon enough, you may be able to breed the mare again that same breeding season.

When you know your mare is pregnant

- Once the mare is confirmed in foal, the vet will perform a Caslicks procedure on her if necessary (see page 7).
- Read this book cover to cover! Pay special attention to chapter 3, "Red-Flag Foaling Problems."

Throughout pregnancy

- Maintain a regular hoof-care program.
- Maintain a regular deworming program. Read labels and be careful to use only products that are safe for pregnant mares.
- Maintain proper nutrition to ensure that the mare and her growing fetus have the necessary vitamins, minerals, protein, and calories.

5 to 6 months before due date

- Schedule an appointment with your vet to update all necessary vaccinations (see page 5).

3 months before due date

- Adjust mare's feed ration to accommodate the critical nutritional requirements of the last trimester (see page 5).

6 weeks before due date

- Schedule appointment with your vet to give mare booster shots of all recommended vaccines anytime within 4 to 6 weeks of foaling.
- Gather foaling supplies and make sure you have everything in one place (see page 13).
- Prepare foaling area (see page 7).
- Start watching the mare closely for any physical changes (see page 11) that signal she is getting closer to foaling. Keep her in a paddock or stall at night where you can check on her easily.
- If she usually lives outside but you plan on having her foal in a stall, now is a good time to start keeping her in the barn at night so she gets used to it.

4 weeks before due date

- Deworm mare for the last time before foaling.
- Have vet open the Caslicks if the mare has one (see page 7).
- Begin using the foaling alarm system if you have decided on this method. Be sure all batteries, transmitters, and receivers are working properly.
- Post a list of emergency numbers by a fully charged phone (see page 11).
- If she will be foaling at a foaling farm, move your mare now (see page 7).

1 to 2 weeks before due date

- If you plan to foal indoors, thoroughly clean and disinfect the foaling stall (see page 9).
- Make sure lighting in foaling area is not too bright.
- Wash the mare's udder (see page 11).
- Check the mare's udder for changes that signal impending foaling (see page 11).
- Watch for changes in attitude; these may signal impending foaling (see page 11).
- Notice when the muscles over the croup and tail head soften and relax.
- Watch for the dense white or off-white mucus plug to be passed. This usually occurs within 72 hours of foaling.
- If her manure is hard and dry, it may be helpful to give the mare a bran mash (see page 44 for recipe), or to wet down her normal feed the day before she foals.

Just before foaling

- Make sure the stall has plenty of fresh bedding.
- Remove water buckets and feed tubs.
- Keep foaling area undisturbed. Observe from outside the stall unless the mare needs help.

2

Your Foal Arrives!

The day you've been waiting for is finally here. Your foal will soon make his grand entry into the world. Ideally, the foaling stall or pen has remained empty until just before the mare nears delivery. This way you always have a clean area ready for the big moment.

When signs indicate the mare is very close to foaling (see box), remove all buckets and feed tubs from her stall or pen. These will just get in the way and can become obstacles for the mare, foal, and any helpers.

It is important to know that your mare may go through most or all of the first stage of labor without your knowledge unless you are paying attention.

"Leaking Milk" Prior to Foaling

Although the mare's udder can begin to fill out as early as four to six weeks before she foals, it will typically appear full and heavy as the she gets closer to foaling. Once you notice that she is "making a bag," check the mare's udder morning and evening as this can give you a good indication of the approaching birth. On occasion, milk will literally stream from the

Signs of Labor

A mare may show some or all of these signs as she gets close to foaling:

- Milk leaking or streaming from udder
- "Wax" on teats
- Walking straddle-legged
- Restlessness
- Pacing the stall
- Pawing and/or lifting hind legs (indicating discomfort)
- Sweating
- Looking at her sides
- Swishing her tail vigorously
- Kicking at her stomach
- Passing small amounts of manure and/or urine frequently
- Lying down and getting up repeatedly
- Edema (swelling) in front of udder along the lower belly

mare's teats and this is generally taken as a sign that she will foal very shortly.

If the mare begins leaking a considerable amount of colostrum before foaling, contact your veterinarian. If she leaks for several days and still hasn't foaled, she may lose all her valuable colostrum (see page 8), so talk to the vet about obtaining frozen replacement colostrum from a farm that banks it.

Getting Down to Business

Once it is obvious that your mare is about to foal, you can wash her hindquarters with warm water and a mild soap. Don't interrupt her, however, if she has actually begun foaling.

Your veterinarian probably won't be present for the delivery unless problems develop, but you should have an experienced horse person familiar with foaling at hand or on call.

Edema, or swelling, along the lower belly may occur shortly before foaling.

Foaling: Stage One

During the first stage of foaling, the mare will show vague or obvious signs of cramping as the foal moves into position for birth. A mare can proceed to stage one, then "shut down" if she doesn't feel safe or relaxed. In the foaling area, create a quiet atmosphere without bright lights. You don't want other horses moving about or other activity that could bother your mare. Until her water breaks, she has the ability to postpone foaling if she is nervous or unsettled.

The mare may lie down and stand up frequently during stage one to reposition the foal. Before the foal moves into the birth canal, it is actually upside down. By rolling, the mare helps the foal move into the desired "diver's position," in which its spine is aligned with its mother's spine.

Stage one may last just an hour or two or as long as ten hours and still be considered in the normal range.

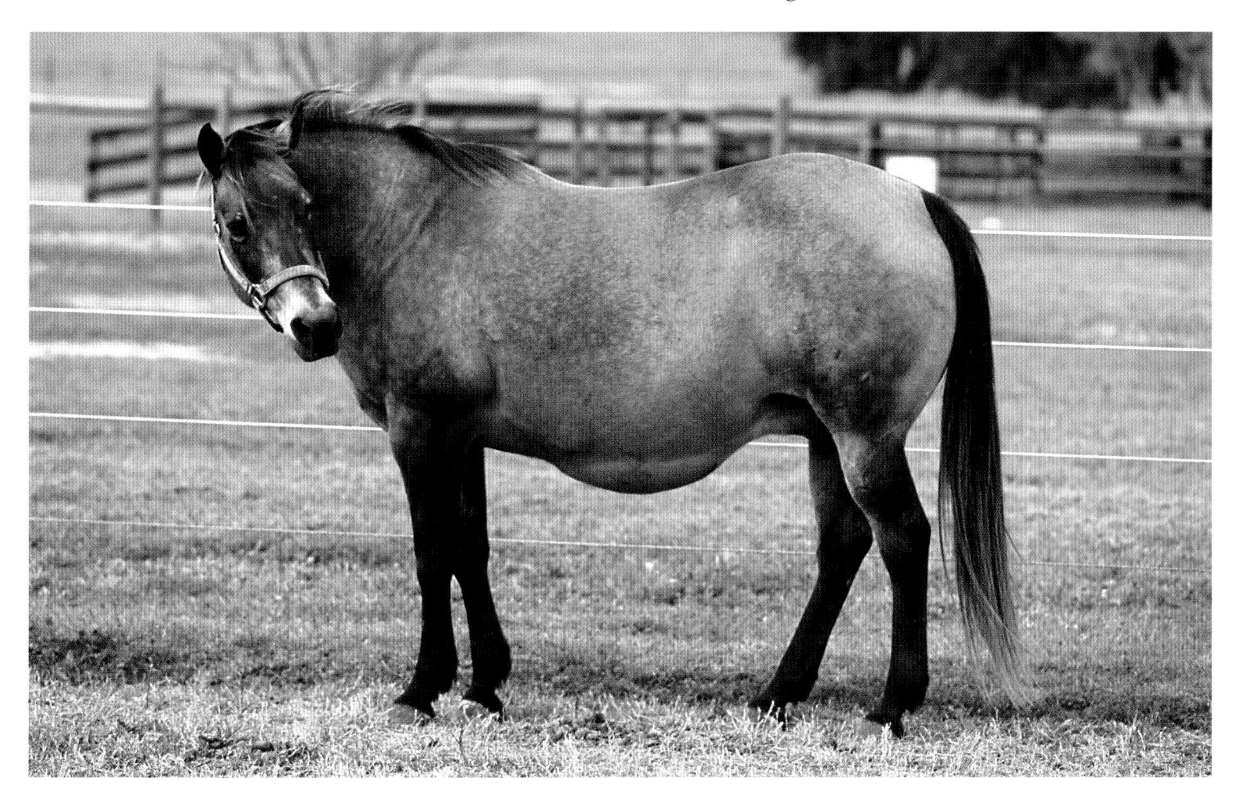

Wrapping the Tail

Some owners wrap the mare's tail to keep it clean and out of the way while the foal is being born. If your mare has never had her tail wrapped before, this process could aggravate or annoy her while she is in active labor. If you want to use a tail wrap, practice wrapping once or twice before the due date to make sure it doesn't bother her.

Ask your vet or an experienced horse person to show you how to wrap a tail. Roll gauze or a plain bandage will work fine, but don't use a self-adhesive elastic wrap: if you wrap it too tight, it can cause serious damage to the tail.

Starting at the top of the tail, use roll gauze or a bandage with Velcro to wrap the tail snuggly but not too tight. Cover the tail at least to where the bone ends. You can braid the rest of the tail or leave it loose.

There is nothing wrong with leaving the mare's tail unwrapped. It *will* get dirty, but you can wash it after foaling.

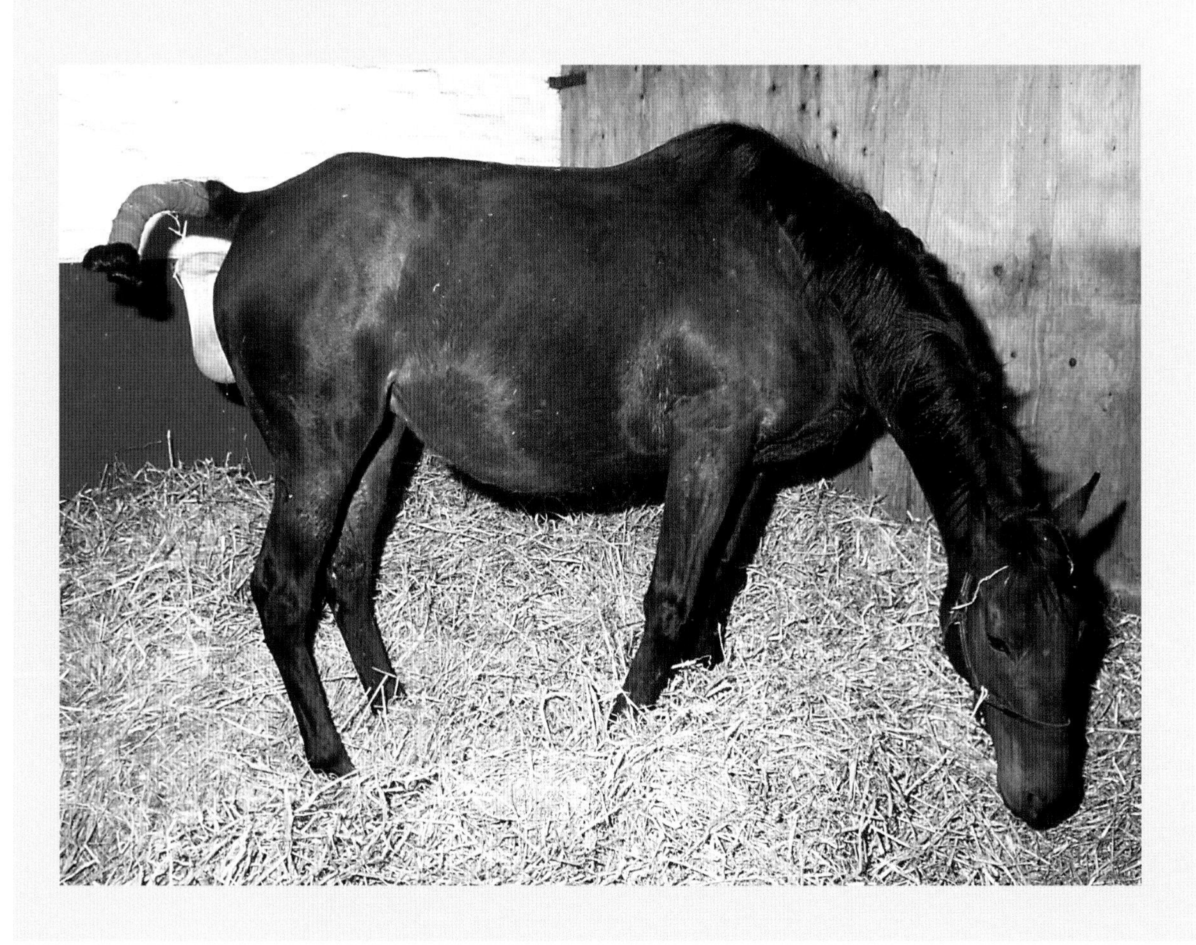

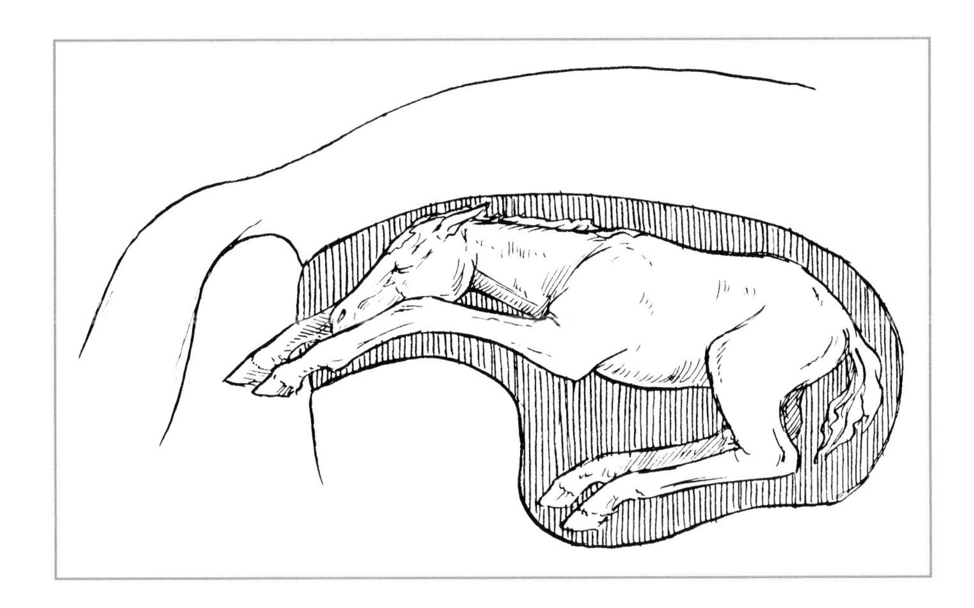

A foal in the normal "diver's position."

Foaling: Stage Two

The second stage of labor begins when the mare's water breaks. This can occur when she is either standing up or lying down. If she is standing up, it may just look as if she is urinating for a long time. What has actually happened is that the membranes of the placenta have been ruptured by the foal's pointed hoof. The several gallons of "water" coming out of the mare are the amniotic fluids in which the foal has been suspended for 11 months.

The breaking water is the most significant sign that the foal is about to be born, after which there is no going back. Once the water breaks, the foal is usually on the ground within 15 to 30 minutes. Pay close attention in case the mare needs assistance, and be ready to take action if required (see page 20). Even with an attended birth, the foal can die because he did not receive the proper aid.

If delivery is progressing normally, however, the mare does not require help. Assisting when the mare doesn't need help can cause bruising and trauma. If the foal is pulled out too quickly, there is the chance of prematurely rupturing the umbilical cord, which can cause hemorrhage.

Your mare will probably lie flat on her side to deliver, so make certain that there is adequate space behind her for the foal to occupy. If she is lying down against the stall wall or a fence, get her up so she will lie down in a better spot and the foal won't be crushed. Occasionally a mare will foal standing up. If your mare starts to foal from this position, you will need assistance so the foal doesn't just fall to the ground.

After the Water Breaks

Soon after the water breaks, you'll see the clear white amniotic sac emerging from the mare's vulva. This bag, which contains the foal, will either break open or stretch through the birth canal intact. Usually, one of the foal's front feet comes first, with the second foot a few inches behind.

It's not unusual at the beginning of the birth process for the foal's feet to appear to be upside down. The foal is typically upside down to start with, and then actually rolls around like a corkscrew as he comes through the birth canal. As long as you are still able to see two front feet and a nose, don't worry. The mare will probably try to reposition the foal if she needs to move it into the desired diver's presentation.

If the foal's front feet and nose are exposed, it means that the amniotic sac has already been broken. Otherwise, the sac covers them. If the sac hasn't broken, now is the time to tear it open and clear it away from the foal's nose. This membrane is tough; you may want to use scissors (carefully), but you can usually poke your fingers through it.

Don't be alarmed if you see thin, clear fluid come out of the foal's mouth and nostrils; after all, he's been swimming in it for the past 11 months. And don't worry if the foal's tongue is hanging out of his mouth before he starts to breathe on his own.

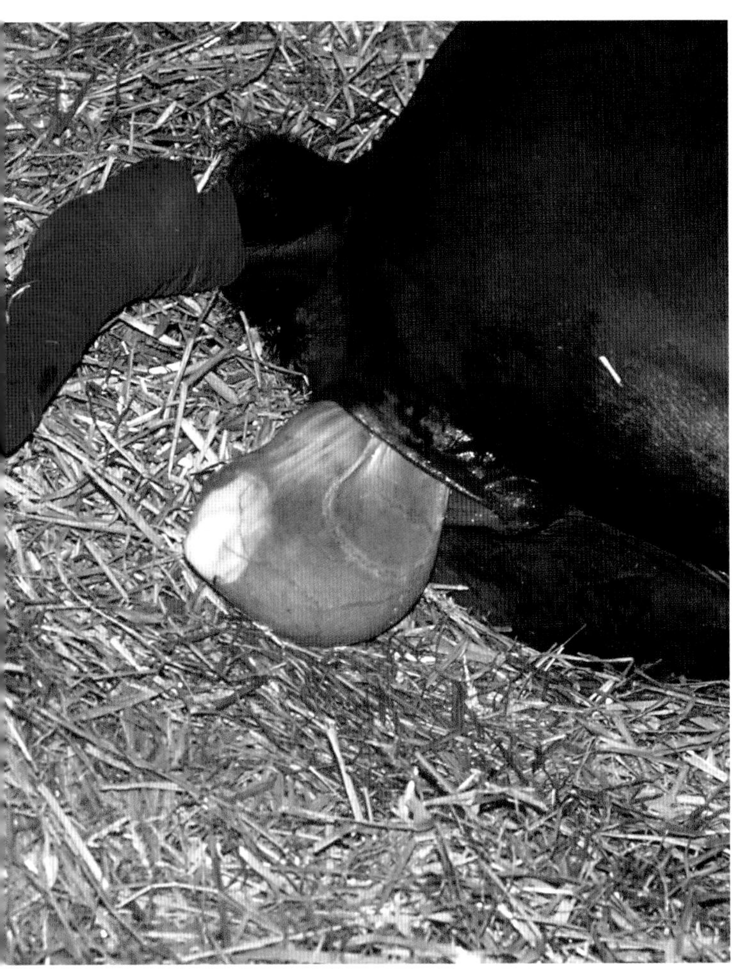

Soon after the water breaks, the white amniotic sac will emerge and you should see one or both of the foal's front feet.

Once the foal is actually in the birth canal, there is pressure on the umbilical cord, but nature has designed the birth process so that this potentially dangerous period is relatively short. Any sustained pinching of the umbilical cord will reduce blood flow and compromise the oxygen supply to the foal.

If you see any presentation other than two front feet and a nose, contact the vet or an experienced foaling person immediately (see chapter 3). Time is precious!

Assisting the Mare

If the foaling is not progressing normally and the mare needs assistance, scrub your hands and arms with warm, soapy water and rinse well. Then follow this procedure.

- Hold the foal's feet in the pastern area above the hooves and below the fetlocks or ankles.
- Pull only when the mare is having a contraction. You just want to maintain firm, steady, downward pressure (toward the mare's hocks) on the foal's legs. The pressure should be out and down.
- When the mare is between contractions, don't actually pull; instead, maintain just enough pressure to keep the foal from slipping back. One average person could probably not pull hard enough to cause any damage, but you should pull *only* when the mare is pushing. You are simply trying to help "shift" the foal so he doesn't get his shoulders or hips caught in the birth canal.
- These few minutes can seem very long, but if the foal is making progress with each contraction, don't try to speed things up. It is common for a mare to rest a few minutes after the hard work of getting out the foal's front feet, head, and neck.

The Birth Process

Labor

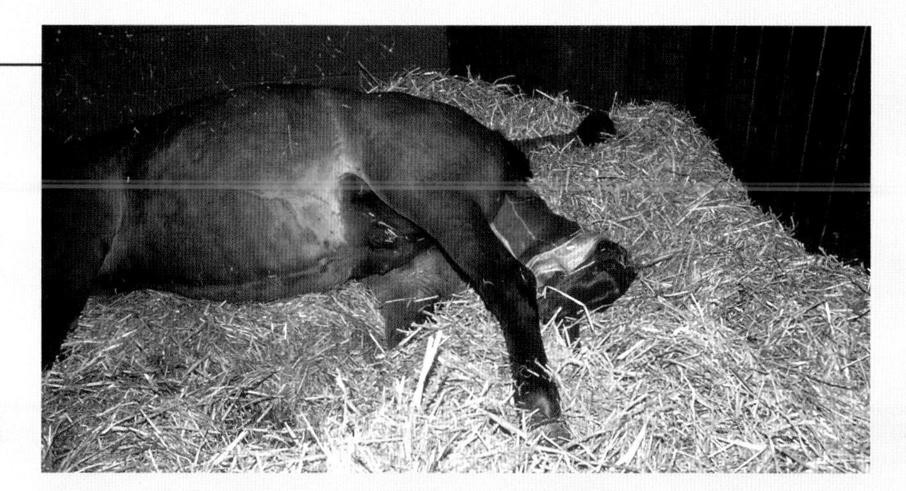

In Stage Two, the mare will typically lie flat on her side, especially for the hard part of pushing the foal's shoulders out. Here, the amniotic sac has already broken.

Delivery

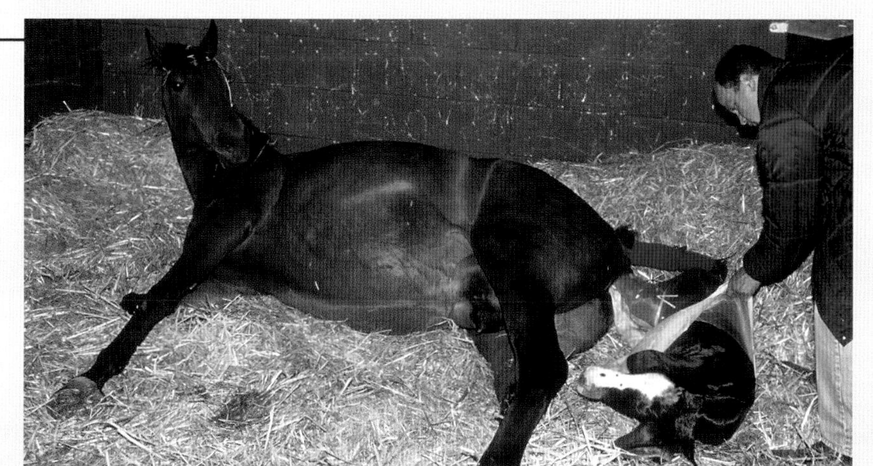

After the shoulders emerge, the rest of the foal slips out with relative ease. The foal's hind legs are usually still in the birth canal at this point.

Newborn

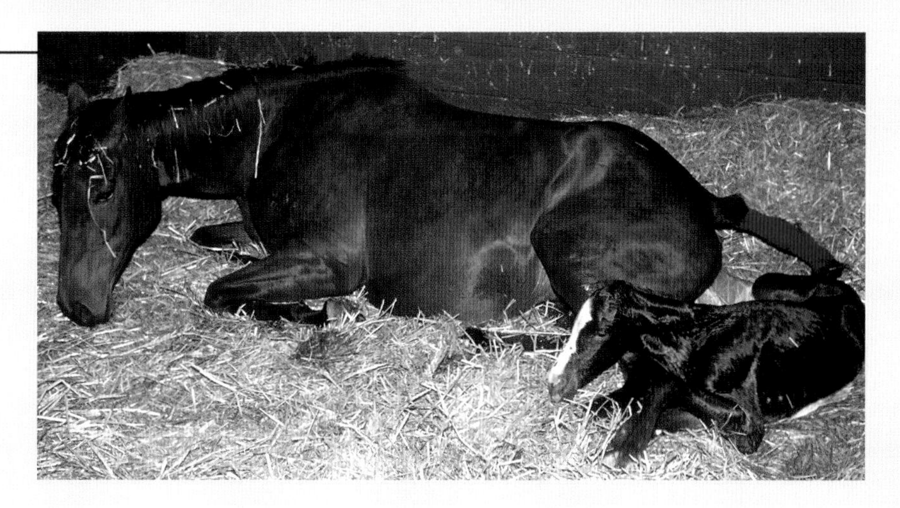

The mare takes a well-deserved rest before getting to her feet. The foal is breathing on his own, but the umbilical cord is still attached and providing him with a flow of enriched blood.

Pushing the foal's shoulders through is the most difficult stage for the mare. Because the shoulders are the largest part of the body to navigate the birth canal, the foal has to actually "slither" out with one foot positioned slightly ahead of the other. After the shoulders emerge, the rest of the foal often slips out with relative ease.

If for any reason the mare gets to her feet when the foal is partially delivered, someone should stand at her head and put a lead rope on her halter so she doesn't turn and sling the foal to the side. Another person holds the foal to keep it from dropping to the ground as it is delivered.

On occasion, a foal's hips may get "locked" in the birth canal. If that happens, you will need to shake and wiggle him free.

Once the foal's body is out, his hind legs will usually remain in the birth canal. Let everyone catch her breath and rest for a few minutes. The mare is often exhausted by this time and probably won't be in a rush to stand up. *Don't be in a hurry to urge the mare to her feet or to break the umbilical cord.* As long as the cord is attached, the foal is receiving a flow of enriched blood. The mare may, at this point, begin paying attention to her foal; she may even nicker to him. The foal's hind legs will usually slip out of the mare as a result of his own struggling. If they have not and the mare acts as though she is going to stand up, pull the foal forward so that his legs are clear of the mare.

Treating the Navel

Ideally, the navel cord will break shortly after birth by the foal's struggles or the mare's. As soon as the cord breaks, apply iodine or properly diluted Nolvasan solution to the stump of the navel. Don't use a spray bottle, sponge, or cotton to put iodine on the navel, and be careful not to splash or spill it on the foal's skin, as it can burn or cause inflammation. Instead, pour the iodine or Nolvasan into a small clean container, such as an empty plastic 60 cc syringe container, a 35 mm film canister, or a plastic pill bottle. Hold the container up against the foal's belly so that the stump of the broken cord is actually dipped into the liquid and saturated, which helps "cauterize" the stump so that a scab forms. This will keep bacteria from entering the foal's system and causing infection or illness. Dip the navel stump several times within the first few days.

Don't pour the unused iodine back into the main container; that will spread germs. Instead, throw away any iodine left in the container you use for dipping.

NEVER use scissors to cut the cord! If for any reason the cord appears unlikely to break, hold it in one hand and pinch firmly with your thumbnail at the narrow fibrous section of the cord, with the palm of your hand close to the foal's abdomen. With your other hand, firmly pull away the cord to cause a "stretch tear." Then treat the resulting stump just as if the cord had broken on its own. The reason you don't use scissors is that this makes a smooth cut, which won't close off and heal as well or as quickly as a stretch tear.

Foaling: Stage Three

Once the foal has been delivered, a mare moves into the third and final stage of the process. Don't be surprised if she acts uncomfortable or appears to be cramping. Often a mare will lie back down and act as if she is foaling again before she passes the placenta.

Before the mare passes the entire placenta, the foaling membranes will be hanging down around her hind legs. If she steps on them while they are still attached inside her, they could tear and cause internal bleeding. If the membranes are hanging so low that they might be stepped on, tie them up out of the way with baling

Foaling ABCs

A — Airway

Make sure the amniotic sac doesn't cover the foal's face and that his **airway** is clear of fluid so that he can breathe.

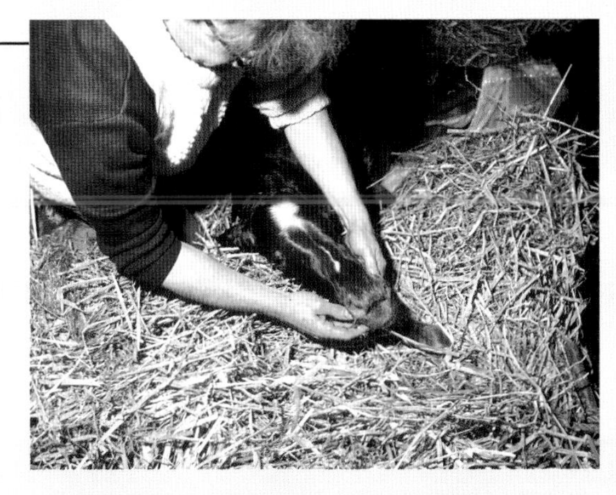

B — Breathing

Make sure the foal is **breathing.** He should be breathing and moving even while his hindquarters are inside the mare. As long as the umbilical cord is attached, the foal is receiving a flow of enriched blood.

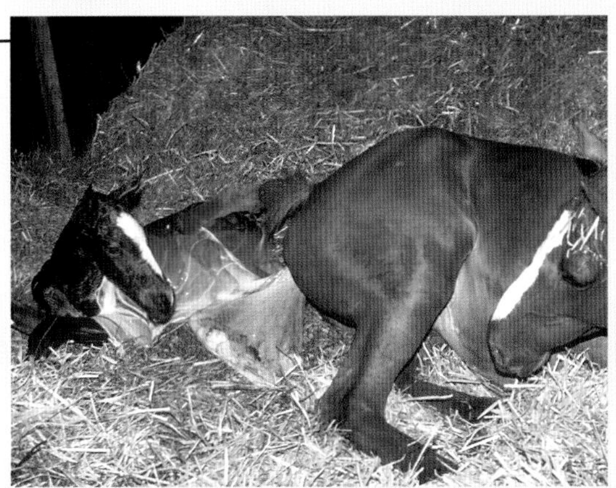

C — Cardiovascular

Stimulate the foal's **circulation** and respiration by vigorously rubbing his whole body with the thick terry cloth towels in your foaling kit. Use a towel to clear any mucus from the foal's ears, eyes, and nose.

Even though the mare is tired from delivery, she will instinctively want to "mother" her newborn. You can dry off the foal by rubbing him with the towel, but be careful not to interfere with the natural bonding that will immediately start between mare and foal.

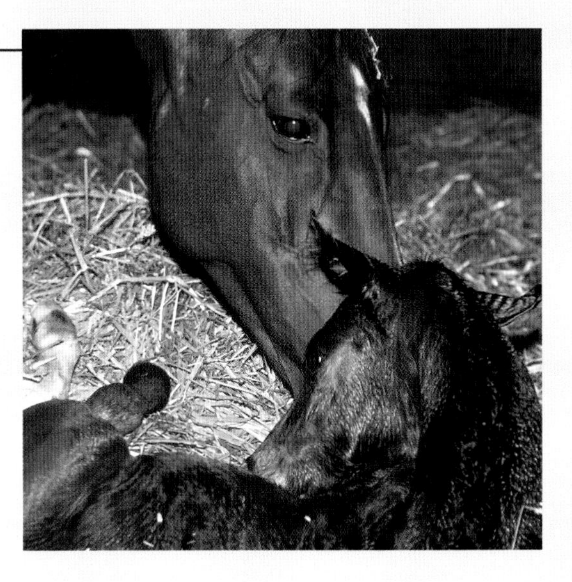

twine from your foaling kit. Tie a loop around the lower section of the placenta, then tie a knot up higher, above the mare's hocks. You can also just tie a knot in the placenta itself, which will be quite slippery, so be very careful not to pull or tug on it.

If your mare is a **maiden** — that is, if this is her first foal — she may bothered by the placental membranes hanging down around her back legs. This is another good reason to carefully tie them up.

Sometimes just the weight of the membranes tied up this way will help to expel the placenta. Do not tie anything heavy to the placenta or try to forcefully remove it to speed things up. This may cause it to tear, and you don't want this to happen. Some of it could remain inside the mare and cause infection. *At no point should you tug or pull on the placenta.*

The mare will usually expel the placenta within an hour after the foal is born. If after two to three hours the placenta hasn't passed and these membranes are still dangling from the mare, call your veterinarian. Upon examining her, he may inject oxytocin, a drug that will cause the uterus to contract and expel the placenta.

Once the foal is born and the placenta is no longer attached to the uterine wall, it becomes a foreign body. If part of the placenta remains inside the mare, she could become toxic. This could lead to cramping, fever, and even **founder** (laminitis), a painful chronic lameness. She

The cord will be broken by the foal struggling or when the mare stands up.

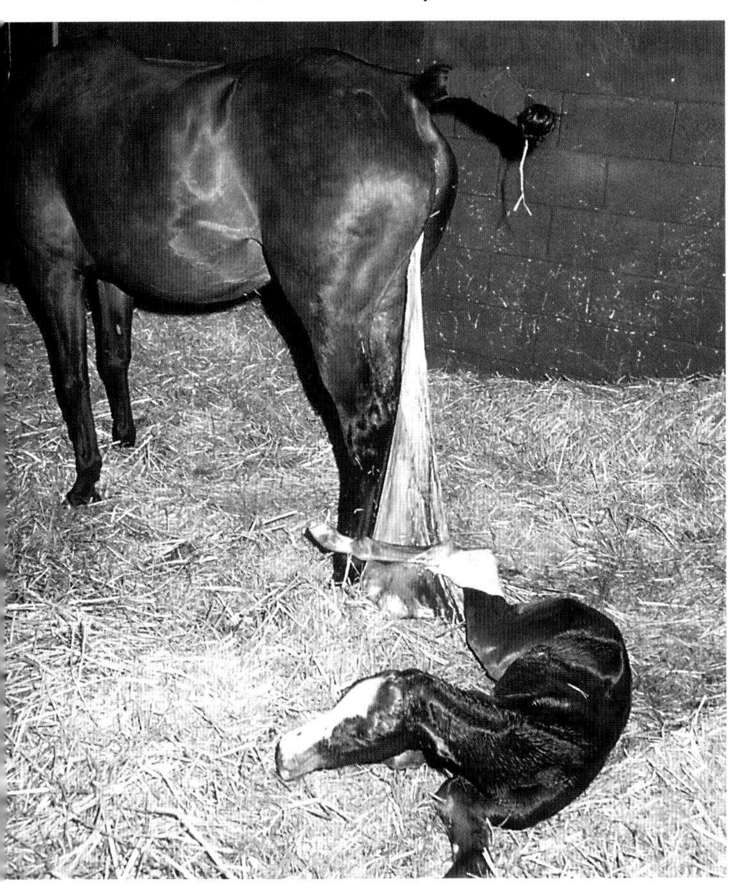

Immediately after the cord is broken, put iodine or Nolvasan on the foal's navel stump.

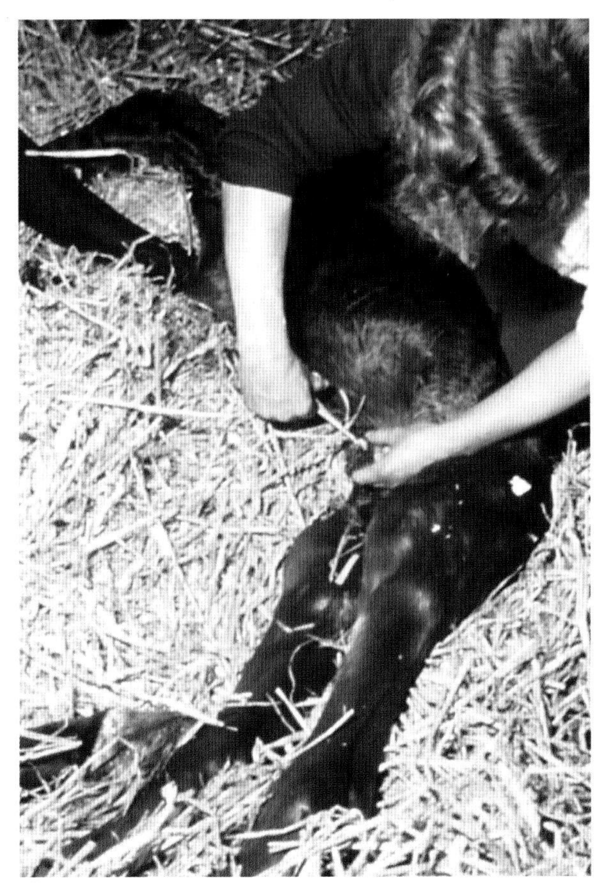

Foaling Words

Amniotic sac (amnion). Innermost membrane of the sac enclosing the foal and amniotic fluids inside the placenta.

Embryo. Term for the unborn foal in the earliest stages of development, through the third month.

Fetus. Term for the unborn foal starting from the fourth month.

Hippomanes. A small, mysterious rubbery tissue mass that is free-floating in the placenta.

Placenta. The organ that develops within the mare's uterus and connects to the fetus by the umbilical cord. It contains the amniotic sac, in which the foal develops.

Presentation. The foal's position in the birth canal at delivery. The easiest presentation is the diver's position, in which the foal is delivered with his nose resting on top of his two front feet.

Umbilical cord. The tough, ropelike cord attached to the unborn foal at the navel that connects it to the placenta. The fetus receives nourishment and oxygen through the umbilical cord, which also removes waste from the unborn foal.

Uterus. The hollow, muscular organ inside the mare in which the foal, contained by the placenta, develops during pregnancy.

might develop a uterine infection, and, in some cases, become infertile. This is why it is so important that the entire placenta be expelled soon after the foal is born.

Once the placenta, also referred to as the **afterbirth,** has been expelled, make sure it is in one piece. If you aren't sure what you are looking for or have any questions, save it in a covered bucket or container for your veterinarian to examine. Spread it out on the floor and examine it carefully. The placenta, which should be reddish in color, should look like a pair of baggy pants. There should be one large tear where the foal broke through. The rest of the placenta should be virtually intact. If you

You can tie up the placental membranes to keep the mare from stepping on them, but *don't* tug or pull on them.

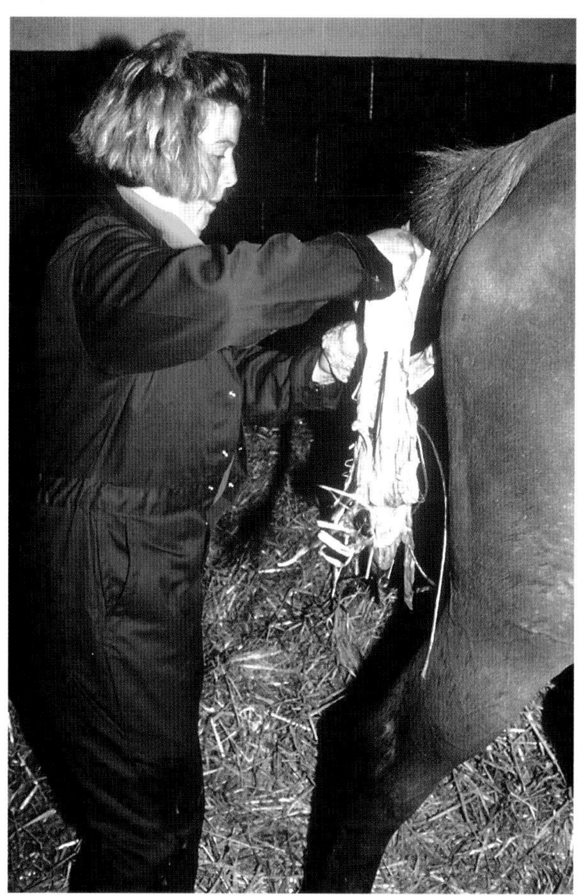

see anything unusual or if pieces of the placenta are missing, tell the vet right away. Missing parts mean that placental fragments have been retained in the mare's uterus. The vet will need to do a postfoaling exam and treat the mare to prevent infection.

You should also see the **hippomanes,** a dark brown or reddish-brown spongy, rubbery mass of tissue that is a dense collection of cells, skin, and hair. Roughly the size of your hand and about one inch thick, this object is free-floating in the placenta, unattached to the foal or the mare. Scientists still don't know the purpose of this mysterious object. Sometimes the hippomanes is expelled during foaling and you will find it when cleaning the stall.

Foal Weight

The weight of an average newborn foal for an average-sized mare is between 95 and 115 pounds.

The hippomanes is a free-floating, spongy mass of tissue in the placenta. This photograph shows its size relative to a quarter.

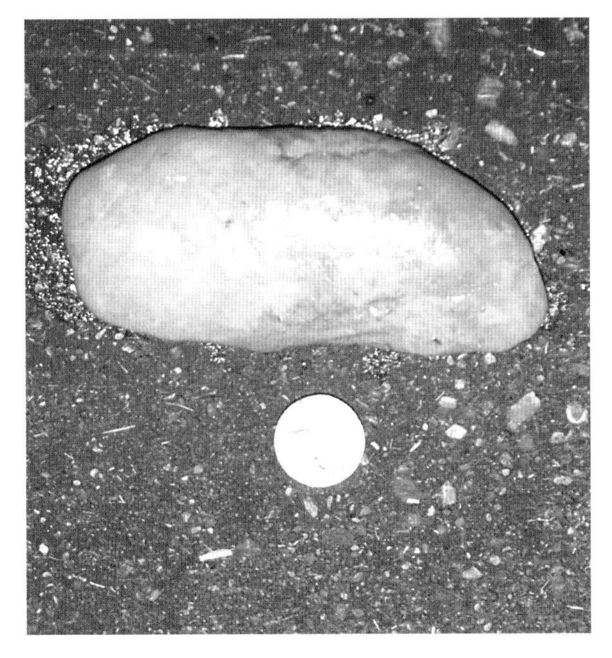

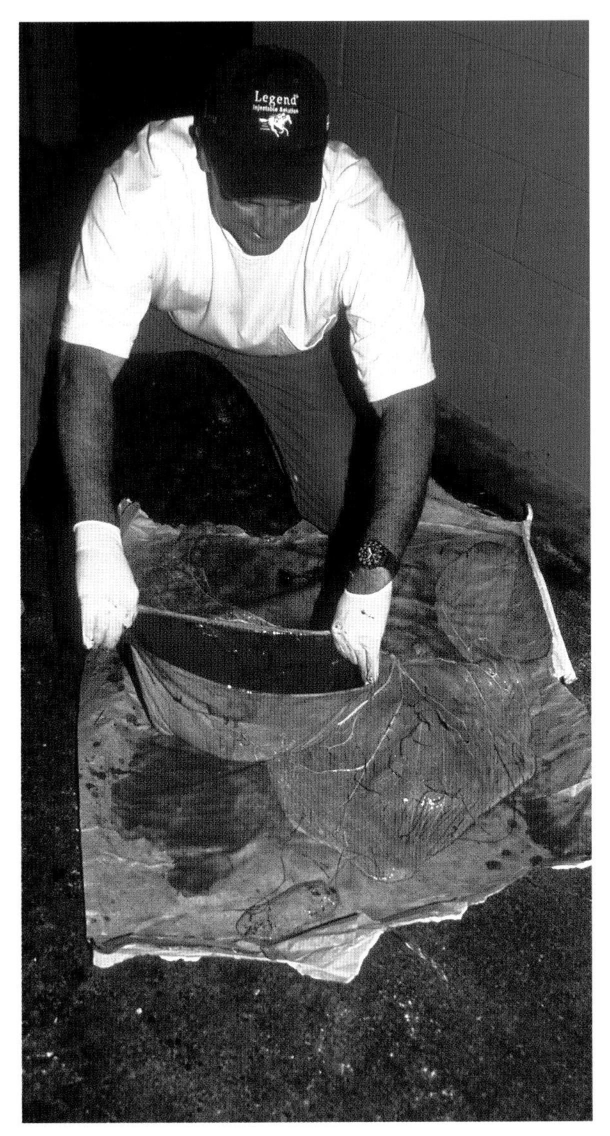

When you examine the afterbirth, there should be only one large tear where the foal broke through.

3

Red-Flag Foaling Problems

What to Do and When to Call the Vet

Mares have been foaling without help for thousands of years. The chances are good that your mare won't need a veterinarian to deliver her foal safely. Of the many mares that foal each year, 95 percent will foal without complications. In all likelihood, your mare will follow the normal foaling pattern.

If things do not follow the step-by-step foaling process (see chapter 2), you will need the assistance of a veterinarian or someone else experienced with foaling. Unlike humans and other animals that can labor for hours and still produce a strong, healthy baby, mares have a much smaller time frame for safe delivery. *Do not delay if you think your mare is having trouble.*

Read this "red-flag" chapter carefully before your mare is due to foal so that you are prepared and can recognize abnormal developments. You probably won't need to act on any of the precautions described here, but because you've been eagerly awaiting your foal for many months, you'll want to be informed.

Most important, if there is any trouble during the foaling, *don't panic.* Instead, focus on being observant so you can describe to the vet or emergency contact person exactly what you see.

Birth Presentation

Presentation describes the foal's position in the birth canal at delivery. The most desired birth presentation is the diver's position, in which the foal is presented with two front feet coming first and its nose resting on top of them. Fortunately, this is the most common presentation. (See illustration on page 19.)

Once the mare's water has broken, if you see any presentation other than two front feet and a nose, consider it an emergency situation and call the vet or your emergency contact immediately. The greatest chance for something to go wrong is during this short part of the birthing process, but at this early stage you also have the best chance for managing problems.

Red-Flag Scenarios

Call your veterinarian *immediately* if you notice any of the following "red-flag" situations. The double red flag indicates an extreme emergency.

Mare Seems Frantic and Tries to Roll

The mare may try to roll during labor because she wants to reposition the foal. Some getting up and down is fine, but there is a difference between the normal behavior caused by painful contractions and the abnormal condition of being frantic. If you think your mare is acting panicky, you're probably right.

Dealing with the Problem

Contact the vet right away.

Progress Stops after Water Breaks

Several minutes pass after the water breaks and there is no sign of the amniotic sac even though the mare is straining.

Dealing with the Problem

Call the vet immediately. While you wait for him, get the mare on her feet and try to keep her walking. This may reposition the foal for a better presentation. Sometimes putting a twitch on the mare's nose while walking her will help slow her contractions and buy a little more time before the vet arrives.

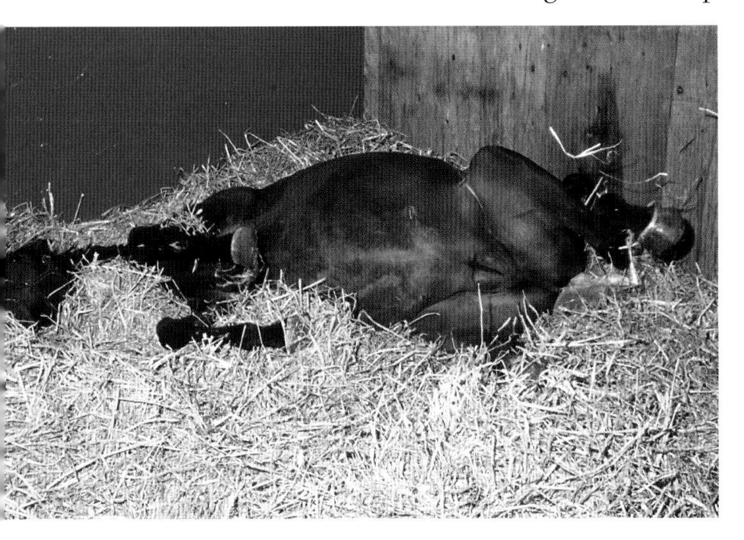

A mare may roll during labor in an attempt to reposition the foal.

Breech Presentation

If the mare's water breaks and she continues in labor with no sac protruding, reach in and check the foal's position, using "clean technique" (see box). If you can feel only the foal's tail and anus, the birth is a breech presentation.

Dealing with the Problem

Contact the vet right away. This requires immediate assistance if there is any hope of the foal surviving. *Do not delay!*

"Clean Technique"

If at any time you need to reach inside the mare to assist with delivery or check the foal's position, you should use "clean technique." This doesn't mean "sterile," but to avoid contaminating the mare, it is important that you follow these steps.

1. Wrap the mare's tail and wash the area around the **perineum** (between the anus and vulva) with water and a mild soap, such as Ivory, then rinse.
2. Wash your hands and arms well.
3. Put on an obstetrical glove from your foaling kit.
4. Use plenty of lubricant, such as K-Y Jelly or methylcellulose (not mineral oil), on the glove whenever you put a hand inside the mare. The mare should never feel "dry" inside.

Back Feet First

If you see feet coming but no nose, check to see if they are front or hind feet. The bottoms of the hooves may be pointed up if they are hind feet or if the foal is still upside down in the normal birthing process before rotating to the desired diver's position. If you aren't sure whether they are front feet or hind, run your hand up one of the foal's legs. If you feel a knee, it's a front leg and the foal is still upside down. If you feel a hock, you know the foal's back feet are coming first.

Dealing with the Problem

Call for help immediately. If experienced help can't get there right away, you will need to assist the mare or the foal may drown in the fluids before he is born.

Get the mare on her feet in the hope that the foal will retreat and be properly repositioned. If the foal continues to emerge in the backward position and the veterinarian has not arrived, you must help deliver the foal by pulling on his legs as the mare strains.

In this position, the umbilical cord will be squeezed or even broken during birth. This signals the foal to start breathing, which is why you have to get the foal out promptly. Once the foal's hips are out, *keep pulling;* otherwise, the foal will inhale fluid and drown.

If the foal was deprived of oxygen during the birth, he may be weak or unconscious. Clear his nostrils as you would normally. Tickle his nostrils with a piece of straw or hay to stimulate breathing. Vigorously rub his body with towels for stimulation. If this doesn't work right away, hold up the foal as high as you can with his head hanging down to let fluids drain out of his airway.

Stained Amniotic Fluid

Amniotic fluid is always clear, so any greenish or yellow staining indicates that the unborn foal was stressed and passed some **meconium** (his first bowel movement) inside the mare.

Dealing with the Problem

Report to the vet any green or yellow stain in the fetal fluids as the foal is being born, even if the delivery is otherwise normal. She will examine the foal carefully after birth and check his

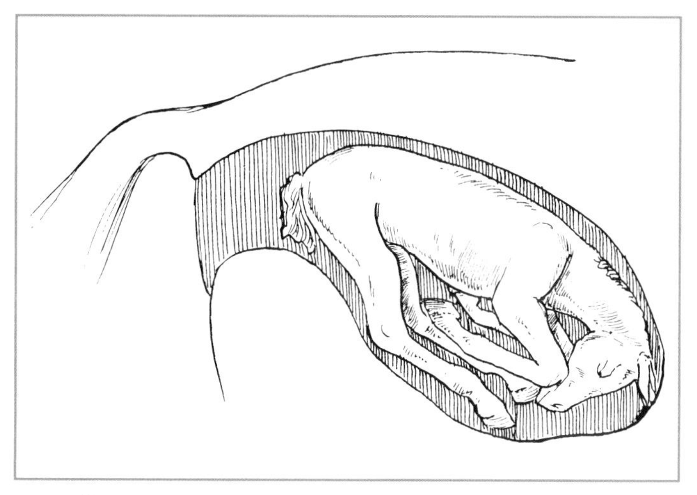

Immediate veterinary assistance is necessary to save a foal in breech presentation.

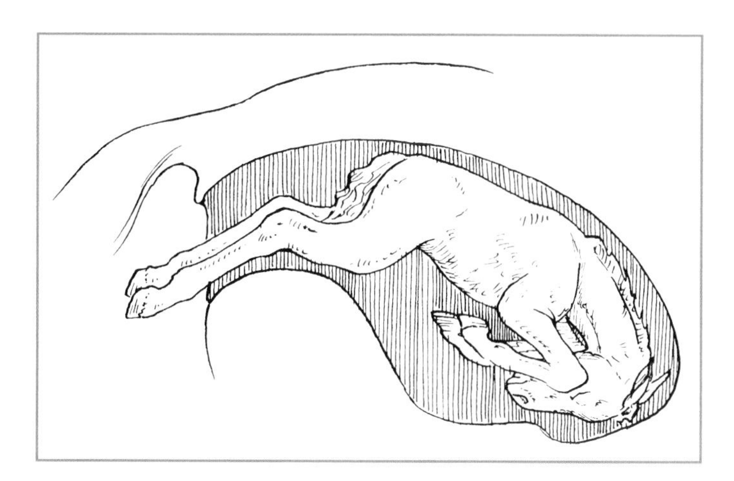

If the foal is coming backward, you must assist the mare, or the foal may drown before he can be born.

lungs. If brain damage occurs due to trauma during birth, there is a danger of aspiration pneumonia and a likelihood of neonatal maladjustment syndrome, in which the foal may have seizures and convulsions and exhibit other neurological signs.

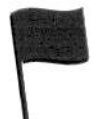

"Red-Bag" Foaling: Placenta Comes First

In the case of **placenta previa,** also known as a **red-bag foaling,** the placenta detaches from the mare's uterus too quickly. Part of the placenta precedes the foal instead of being expelled after the foal is born. (The term *red bag* comes from the appearance of the dark red membrane you will see coming out of the mare first, rather than the white amniotic sac.)

Dealing with the Problem

In a red-bag foaling, it is important to act immediately. If the foal is deprived of oxygen because of the early detachment of the placenta, he is at risk of becoming a "dummy foal," which means that brain swelling develops within the first 24 hours. Any time you suspect the foal may have been deprived of oxygen during birth, call the veterinarian.

Break open the tough placental membrane (you may need to use the scissors in your foaling kit). In a red-bag birth, there will be two "layers" to open: the red bag of the placenta and the smooth white bubble of the amniotic sac, which contains the foal. Locate the foal's head and front feet, and assist the mare with delivery (see chapter 2). Following a red-bag foaling, the vet may want to treat the foal for oxygen deprivation.

Foal Doesn't Breathe

If the foal doesn't start breathing on his own right away, follow the ABCs described on page 23 in chapter 2.

Dealing with the Problem

Make sure the amniotic sac is off the foal's face and that his airway is clear of fluid. Use vigorous stimulation and rub the foal with towels. With the foal lying on his side, block the nostril closest to the ground with your finger and place your mouth against the top nostril. Rhythmically blow air into this nostril (mouth to nostril) until you see the lungs inflate. Once the foal is breathing, he can continue to breathe more easily if he is lying in an upright position on his chest, or **sternum,** rather than flat on his side. Reposition the foal so that he is upright after he is breathing on his own.

Mare Hemorrhages

Occasionally, a mare will rupture an artery or major blood vessel during foaling. **Hemorrhage** happens more often in older mares that have had multiple foals, and can occur immediately after foaling or not until hours later.

In the case of internal hemorrhage, blood will not seep out of the mare's vulva. Be aware of the following symptoms, any of which can signal internal bleeding:

- moderate coliclike abdominal discomfort
- sweating
- continual pawing and general anxiety
- pale, white gums and **sclera** (white part of the eye)

Dealing with the Problem

Caution: If the mare is hemorrhaging, get the foal and any people in the stall out of the way, as she may fall or thrash about. *Keep the foal and his handlers out of harm's way — even a docile mare can become dangerous when she is dying.*

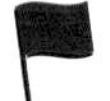

Uterine Prolapse

In some rare cases, the mare will suffer a **uterine prolapse** after foaling. This means that her whole uterus, not just the placenta, is expelled after the foal is born. Call the vet: a prolapsed uterus must be treated immediately in order to save the mare.

Dealing with the Problem

Hold the mare still until the vet arrives. Support the prolapsed uterus with a clean wet sheet or blanket so that its weight does not strain the blood vessels and cause hemorrhage. Three people will be needed: one person holds the mare while the other two support the uterus.

Jaundiced-Foal Syndrome

Jaundiced-foal syndrome occurs when the foal's blood type is incompatible with the mare's and the mother produces antibodies that actually "fight" against her foal's red blood cells. If your veterinarian has any suspicion that this is a possibility, particularly if the mare has borne a jaundiced foal in the past, a neonatal isoerythrolysis (NI) or "cross-match" test can be performed on the mare's blood two weeks prior to foaling. If no NI test has been performed, the only indications of jaundiced-foal

The foal will be able to breathe more easily if he is lying in an upright position, not flat on his side.

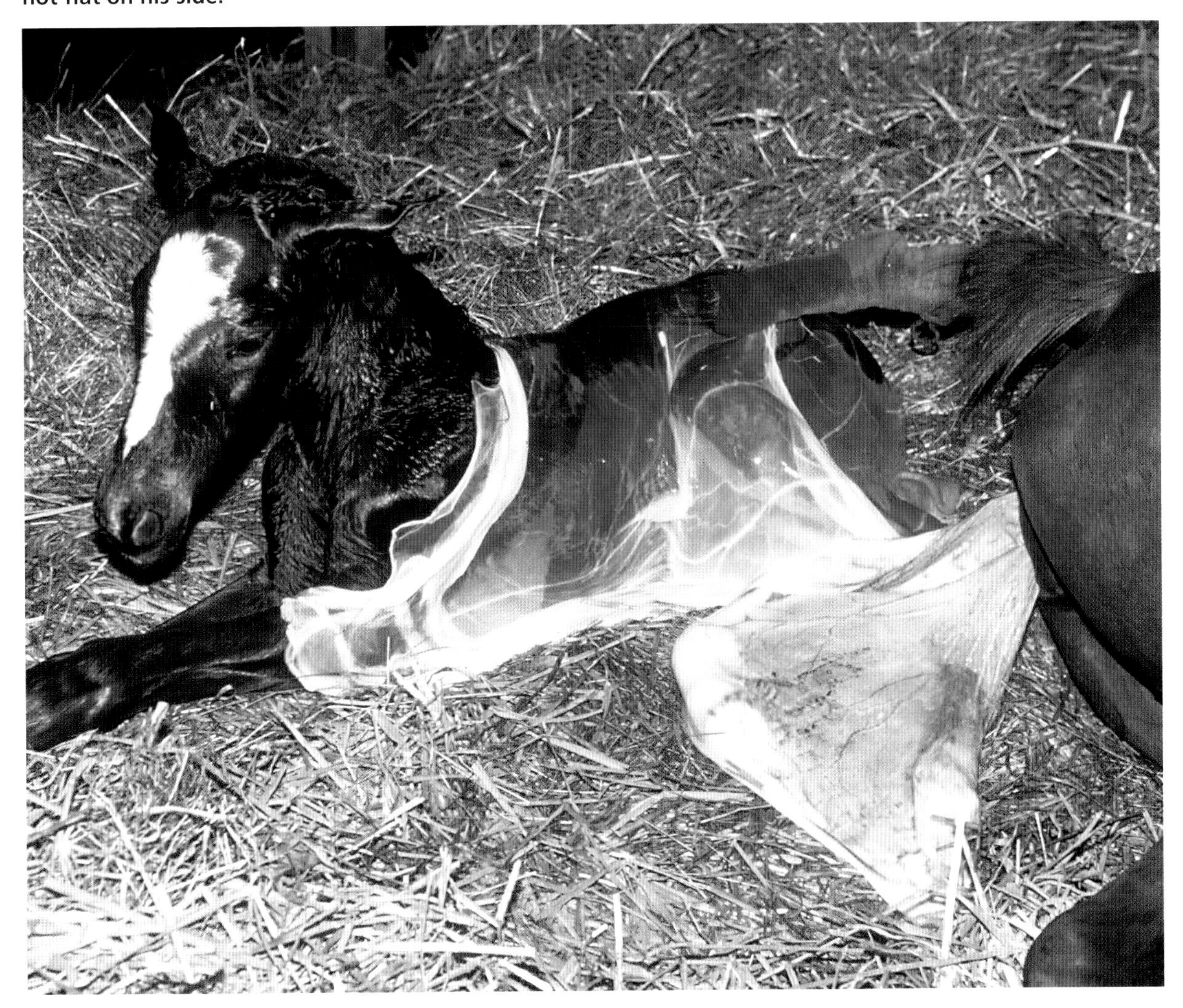

Treating the Navel

If the foal's navel stump bleeds, use your disinfected fingers, a clean clothespin, a rubber band, or an umbilical clamp to stop the bleeding. *Do not try to tie off the cord after it breaks.* Make sure it has been saturated with iodine or Nolvasan solution after it breaks to prevent bacteria from infecting the foal by way of the navel. Dip the navel stump several times over the first few days to be on the safe side.

syndrome are developing clinical signs in the newborn.

If the test is positive, do not allow the newborn to nurse, especially during the first 24 hours, as the colostrum will pass on dangerous antibodies to the foal. Instead, bottle-feed the foal and provide a colostrum supplement. The mare must be milked out frequently by hand to eliminate the undesirable colostrum and encourage milk production. When the foal is with his mother, muzzle him so he cannot nurse until testing shows that negative antibodies are no longer present.

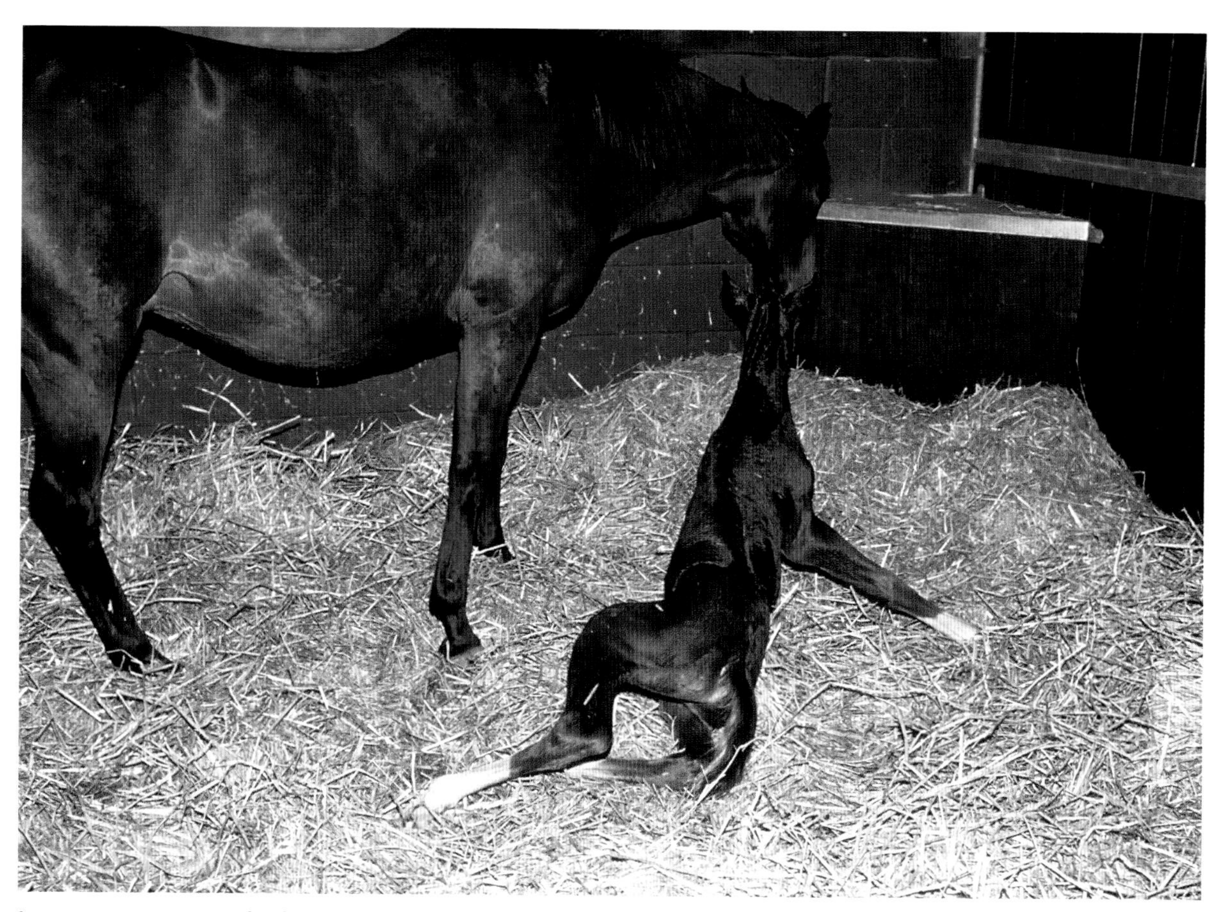

In severe cases, angular limb deformities will interfere with the foal's ability to stand.

Normal Newborn Foal Check

If a newborn foal doesn't fall into these normal ranges, call your veterinarian.

Heart rate: 60–120 beats per minute (should be 80–100 beats per minute by 24 hours old).

Respiration: 40–60 breaths per minute (should be about 30 breaths per minute by 24 hours old). Noticeably shallow, slow, or irregular breathing is cause for concern.

Temperature: 99–102°F. Newborn foals rarely have an elevated temperature, and a below-normal reading is an indication that something serious maybe wrong.

Gums: Should be pink.

Suckle reflex: Should start within 10 minutes of birth.

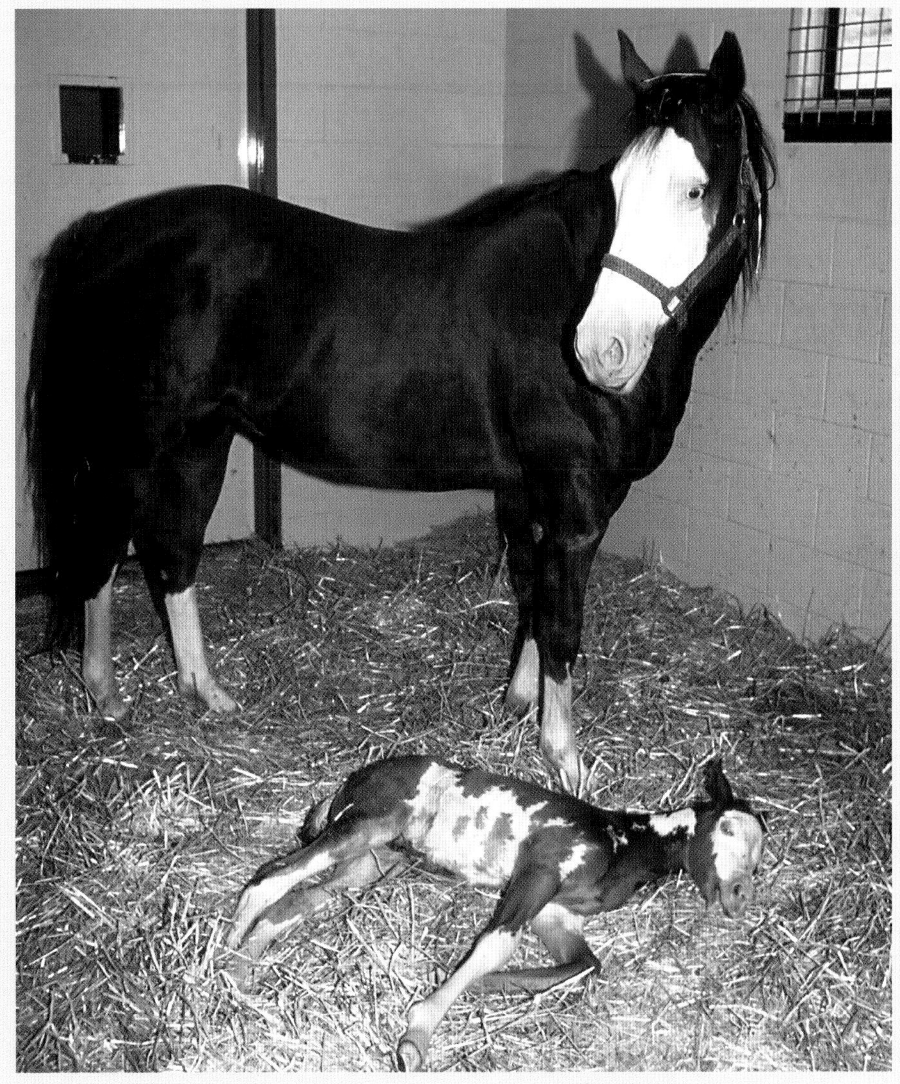

It is normal for a newborn foal to take a nap soon after birth.

Causes for Concern in the Newborn Foal

If you notice any of these symptoms within the first hours or even days, contact the veterinarian.

- Not following mare
- Inability to be aroused or to stay awake
- Loss of interest in nursing or not nursing regularly
- Loss of appetite
- Lack of interest in surroundings
- Depression
- Large amounts of milk on foal's face (from mare dripping milk)
- Milk coming out of foal's nostrils after nursing
- Mare's udder distended (sign of foal not nursing regularly)
- Umbilical abnormalities
- Hot, swollen navel cord or discharge from navel cord (sign of an infected navel cord)
- Increased temperature (may signal developing infection)
- Angular limb deformities or any deviation from normal in either the front or hind limbs; in severe cases, deformities can actually interfere with the foal's ability to stand
- Any swelling in the limbs and especially the joints; some swelling can be normal on foal's first day, but take note
- Difficulty breathing (could indicate fractured ribs caused by the birthing process or from trauma after birth)
- Unusual noises when breathing, such as snorting and rattling
- Inappropriate vocalization: anything other than normal nickering or whinnying
- Difficulty urinating or straining to urinate with little output resulting (could indicate a ruptured bladder)
- Abdominal bloating (an indication of a ruptured bladder, typically noticed three to four days after foaling, and more common in colts than in fillies)
- Blood in stool, difficulty passing stool, or straining after diarrhea
- Abnormal posture or behavior, any straining, any difficulty getting up
- Rolling on his back with head and neck outstretched while upside down (could indicate impacted meconium or constipation)
- Arched "squirrel tail" (a sign of impaction or constipation)
- Tilted head with flickering eyes (not to be confused with blinking), called nystagmus (a sign of seizure)
- Cloudiness of the eyes
- Dilated pupils, foal bumping into things
- Congenital abnormalities of the eye
- Reddened streaks in the sclera (white part of the eye)
- Bright green pupil in one or both eyes (serious sign of septicemia)
- Inverted eyelids (a condition in which the hair on the eyelid actually scratches the cornea, causing ulceration; can be present at birth)

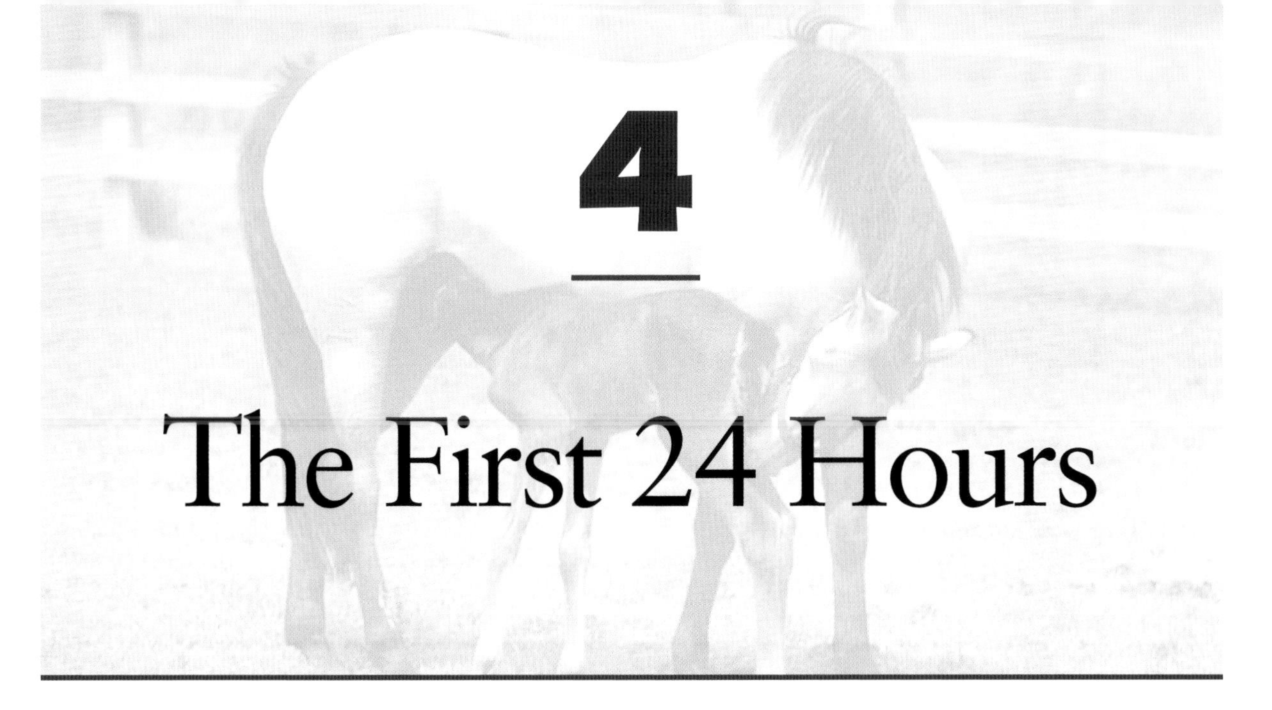

4

The First 24 Hours

Congratulations! The long-awaited day is finally here and your foal has arrived. Now what?

The first 24 hours after birth are extremely important for your foal's healthy start in life. The foal's **dam,** his mother, also needs attention to be sure she is doing well after the hard work of delivering her foal.

First Priorities

Her new baby is the mare's main focus, and she will behave like a new mother by nickering, nuzzling, and licking him. It isn't unusual for her to act overly protective during the first couple of days. A normally quiet mare may show some aggression even to people she knows. She may try to position herself protectively between you and the foal. This behavior should decrease or disappear as the mare relaxes and the foal is nursing regularly.

The new foal's primary concern is finding his first meal. He instinctively knows that he must somehow get to his feet and find something to eat!

Precious Colostrum

Colostrum, the first fluid produced by the mare's udder, is critical because it contains antibodies that will protect the foal during the first several months of life, until his own immune system develops. The mare's udder contains colostrum for only the first 24 to 48 hours after birth. It is then replaced by regular milk, which will nourish the foal but does not contain the same valuable antibodies. As the foal's gut can absorb these protective antibodies only for the first 24 hours after birth, the importance of getting colostrum into the newborn during this short period cannot be overestimated. Quality colostrum is sticky, slightly yellowish, and creamy in consistency.

Wash the Udder

Even though you washed the mare's udder a few days before she foaled, it's crucial to clean it again before the foal nurses for the first time. Foaling fluids, blood, dirt, and manure can easily contaminate the udder during the foaling process. As the foal fumbles around trying to find his lunch, he can ingest bacteria from the mare's body, causing infection.

Clean the mare when she stands up after foaling and before the baby nurses for the first time. Have someone hold her close to the foal so she can see him. Carefully wash her udder and hindquarters with warm water and soap, rinse well, then dry the area with a clean towel before allowing the foal to nurse.

First Nursing

A normal foal will try to stand up within the first hour after birth, often within 15 or 20 minutes. His long legs will present an awkward challenge and he is sure to fall numerous times before he finally stays on his feet. Rubber padding on the stall walls or banking the walls with straw or bedding hay will help cushion those first stumbling attempts. The foal will learn to brace himself and stand, but don't be afraid to intervene and help him balance if he's about to tumble into a wall.

Once the foal is fairly steady on his feet, he will search for his dam's udder. Foals have a strong suckle instinct and may try to suck anything that comes in contact with their mouths. Some experienced mares will position themselves helpfully and use their nose to nudge the foal into place. If the foal has trouble locating the udder, you can gently guide him into position, but make sure someone else is holding the mare's head so she doesn't move around and knock into you or the foal. The mare's udder is usually uncomfortable in the beginning because it is tight and full of milk, and a young or nervous mare may need the reassurance of someone standing at her head while someone else assists the foal as he nurses for the first time.

Don't expect the foal to nurse for very long. He may take only a few swallows before he lies down to rest. The important thing is that he does "latch on" and swallows the vital colostrum he needs for protection against

The normal foal tries to stand to nurse within the first hour after birth.

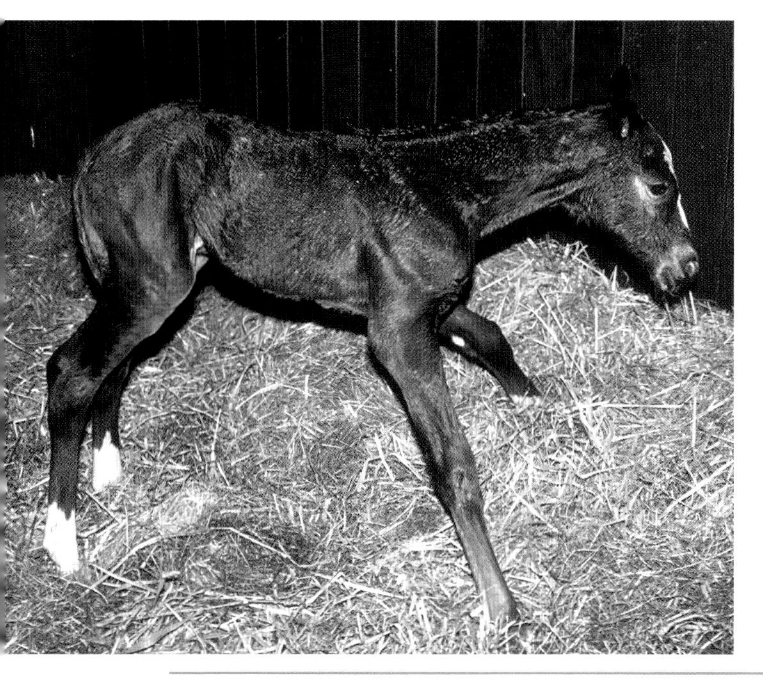

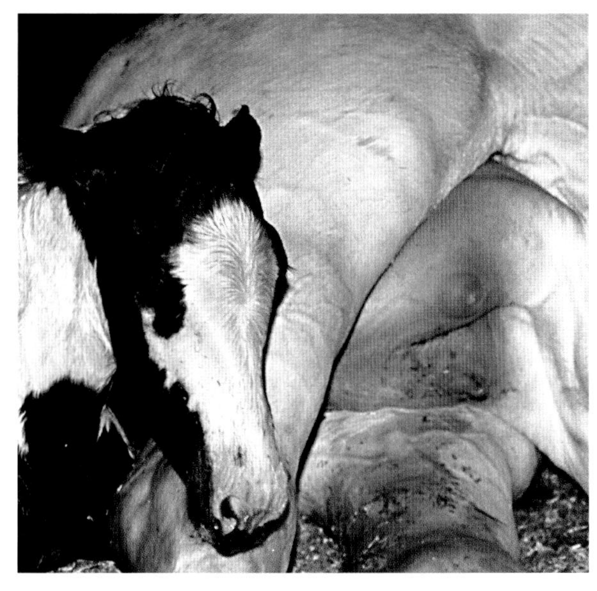

The mare's udder is typically contaminated with foaling fluids, dirt, and manure during the foaling process and should be cleaned before the foal nurses for the first time.

bacteria and disease. After the big effort of nursing for the first time, he will likely take a short nap, but it won't be long before he is back on his feet and nursing again.

Once the mare and foal are resting comfortably, take a few minutes to remove the wet and bloody areas of straw or bedding hay in the stall, then add some fresh, dry bedding.

Bottle-Feeding the First Meal

Very occasionally, the vet will advise you to give the foal his first feeding from a bottle before he even tries to stands up. For example, if there has been a problem with other foals becoming ill, the vet may want you to introduce some of the mare's colostrum immediately. This isn't usually necessary, but discuss the possibility with your vet before foaling so you will be prepared.

If you use frozen colostrum, don't boil or microwave it — that destroys the valuable antibodies. Instead, just thaw the bottle or bag of colostrum in a bowl or bucket of warm water, and then bottle-feed it to the foal (see page 39). Newborn foals should receive at least 1 to 1½ pints of colostrum.

Feeding the foal his first small meal from a bottle won't discourage him from standing up and nursing from the mare later. In addition to getting those important antibodies into his system, bottle-feeding will give him energy and has a laxative effect, which will help him pass the meconium, his first stool.

Navel Care

It's critical to stop any bleeding from the foal's navel stump after the cord has broken. It's a good idea to have an umbilical clamp handy in your foaling kit, just in case. Attach the clamp to the navel stump close to the foal's belly to stop any bleeding. If you don't have a clamp, use a wooden clothespin or rubber band. Make sure the navel stump has been saturated with iodine or Nolvasan solution. If you use Nolvasan, dilute at 1 part Nolvasan to 4 parts water. If you aren't positive that the stump was thoroughly treated as soon as the cord broke, treat it again now. This is important to prevent bacteria from causing infection.

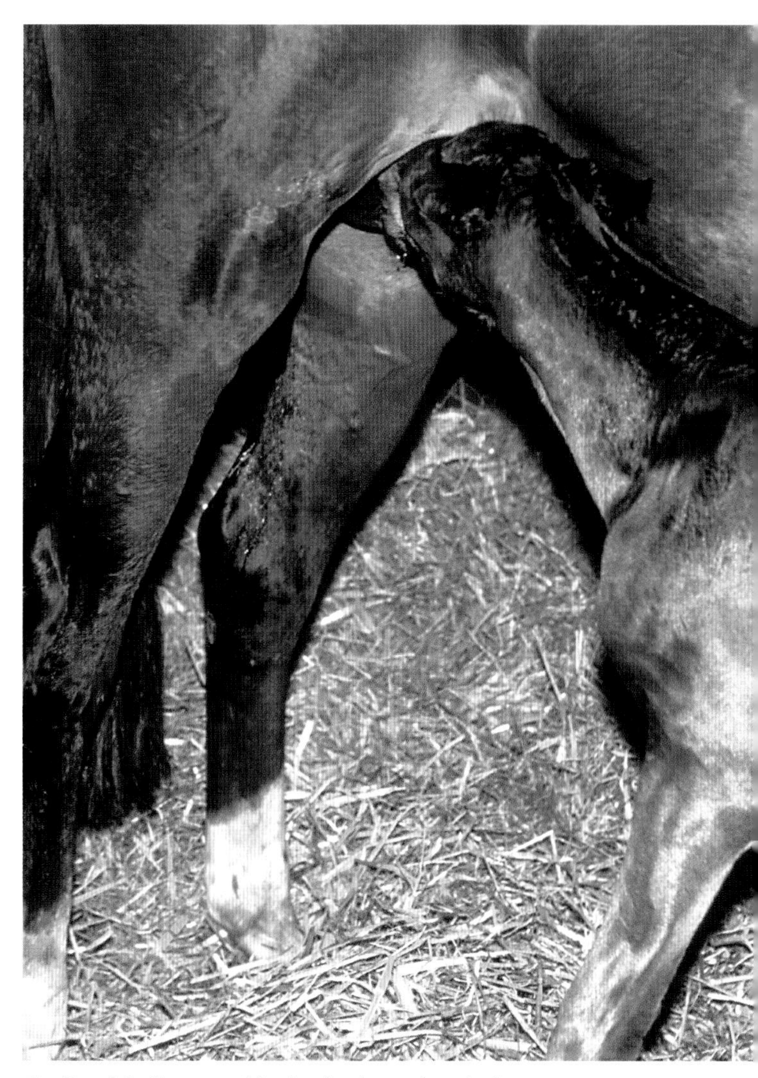

Finding his first meal is the foal's main mission once he has gotten to his feet.

Research has shown that sooner is better when it comes to getting colostrum into the newborn. If the foal receives just 4 to 6 ounces of colostrum as soon as he starts trying to suckle, the chances of septicemia, an infection in the bloodstream (see page 41), are drastically reduced.

Most foals will stand within an hour of birth and then nurse within an hour of standing. The foal should nurse on his own within two hours after birth, but if he hasn't nursed after four hours, *contact your vet immediately. Never wait until the new foal actually looks sick.*

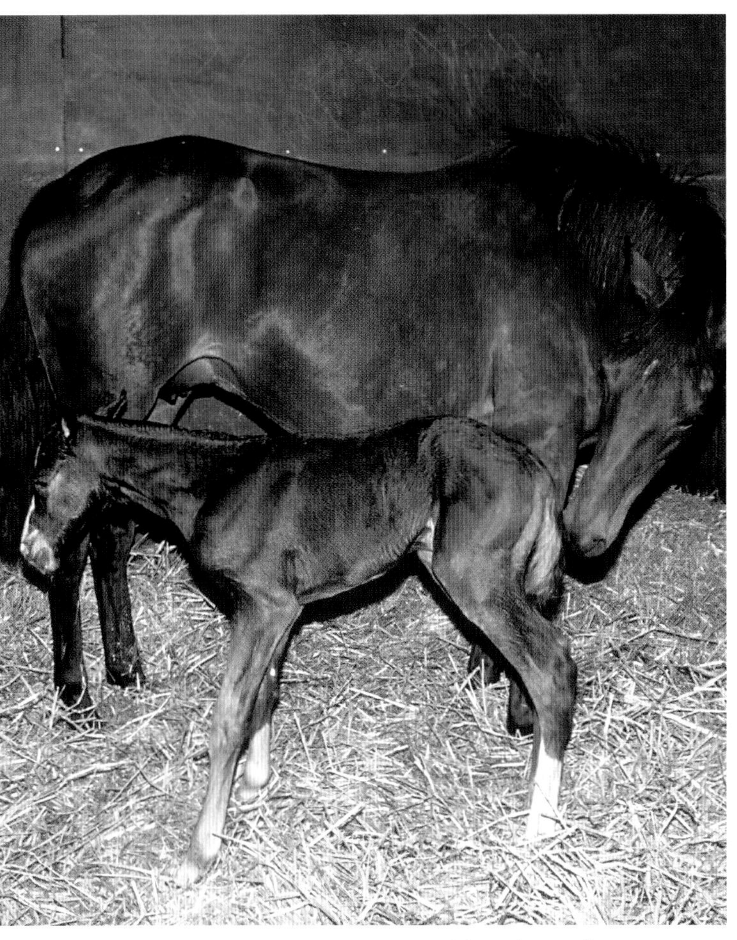

Some mares will try to position themselves to help the foal find the udder. If the foal is having difficulty doing this, you can help guide him into position.

Foal Feet

While your foal is lying down and resting, take a close look at his feet. Instead of the clearly defined V-shaped frog and hard sole seen on an older horse, the bottoms of the newborn's hooves have soft, flexible layers of feathery-looking tissue. This is normal. In just a few days the foal's feet will toughen up and you'll be able to see the frog clearly defined. It would be tough on the mare during delivery if the unborn foal's hooves were as hard as an adult horse's. Nature has designed the foal's hooves so that they don't harden until after birth.

Unlike an adult horse's hoof, a foal's hoof has soft, feathery layers of tissue.

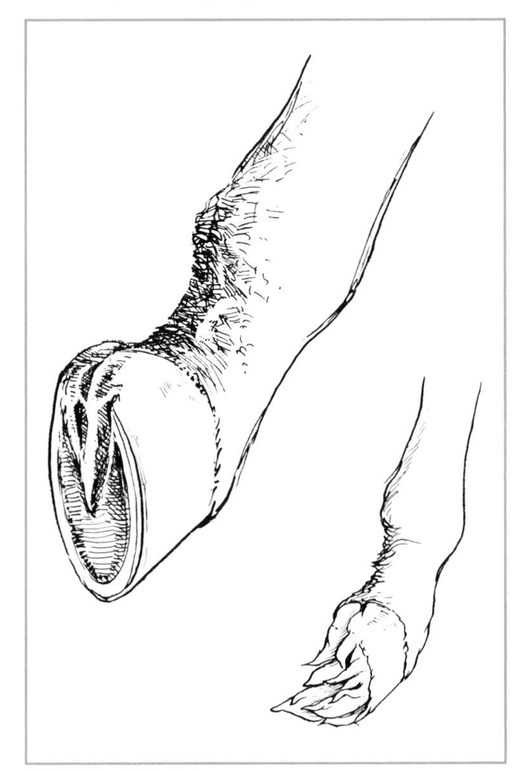

If the foal seems especially weak, the vet may choose to tube-feed the first meal by passing a nasogastric tube through the foal's nose into the stomach. This simple procedure allows the foal to receive the benefits of colostrum immediately without any effort on his own.

Sometimes the foal needs the vet's help only with this one tube-feeding to gain enough strength to stand and nurse on his own. In situations where the foal is still weak, he may require additional tube-feeding, or bottle-feeding and/or your assistance, to help him stand and nurse from the mare the first few times. If for any reason, the vet has to come out to tube-feed the foal, keep in close contact with her so she knows how the foal is doing in case he needs further assistance.

Normal Newborn Foal Activities

It's vital to know what to expect from your newborn foal. If there are any problems, early intervention on the part of your veterinarian can be critical, as a sick foal can deteriorate within hours. On the positive side, a sick foal that receives proper medical attention can rebound quickly.

Nursing

A new foal will nurse frequently throughout the day with short naps between sessions. As with human babies, eating and sleeping are routine in the early days of life.

Bottle-Feeding

To bottle-feed the foal, use a standard plastic baby bottle. Attach a regular infant nipple but enlarge the hole slightly.

1. Wash the mare's udder.
2. While someone holds the mare,collect some colostrum by gently squeezing the teats to express a few streams of fluid into the baby bottle. You need only 4 to 6 ounces.
3. Put the nipple directly into the foal's mouth. Most foals will try to suckle even before they manage to stand up and should drink readily from a bottle.

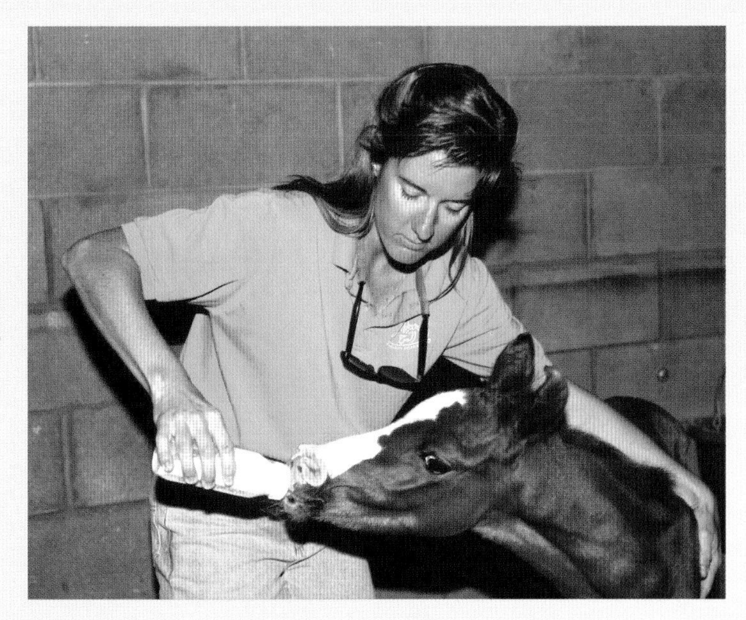

The 1-2-3 Rule

On average, the typical healthy foal should stand within **one** hour of birth, nurse within **two** hours of birth, and pass the meconium within **three** hours of birth.

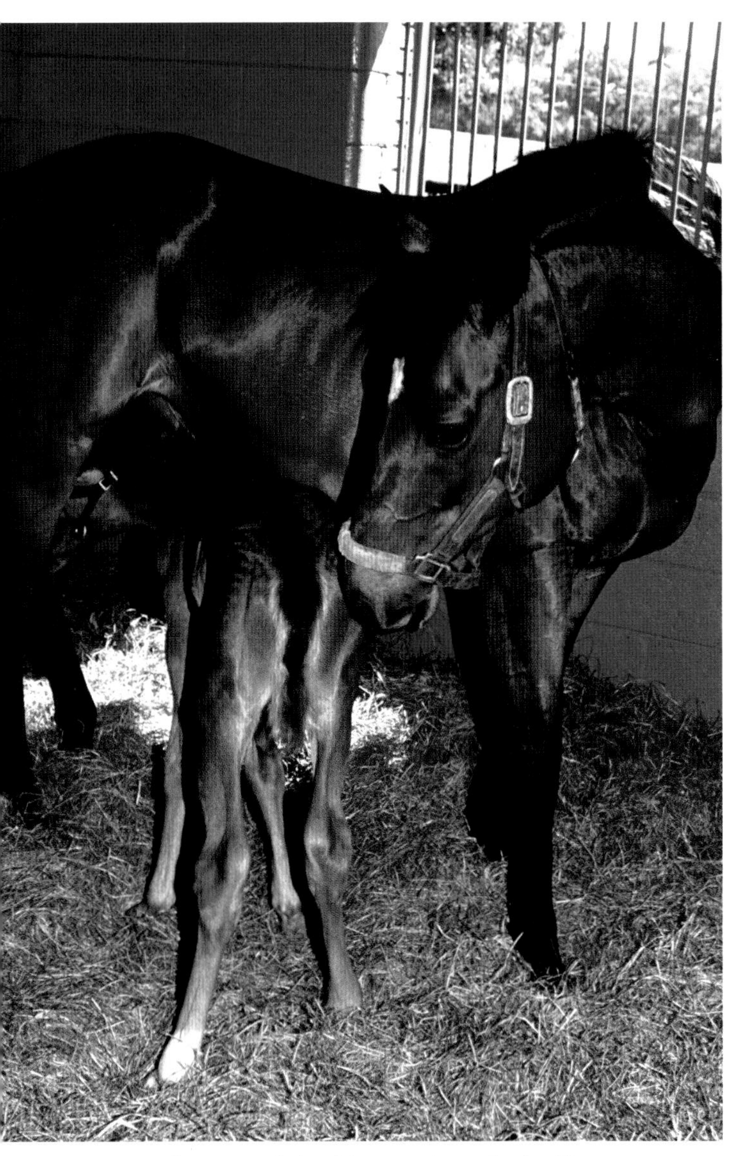

The normal, healthy newborn foal will nurse every time he wakes up, usually every 30 minutes to an hour.

A healthy foal will nurse five to seven times an hour when awake. He will nurse every time he wakes up from sleeping, usually every 30 minutes to an hour. The average young foal will drink roughly 2 gallons of milk throughout the day, or 12 to 20 percent of his body weight.

A normal nursing pattern is the first indicator that your foal is healthy. The foal's nursing also stimulates the mare's uterus to contract, which in turn helps her to expel the placenta more quickly.

Keep an eye on the mare's udder. After 24 hours, when the foal has figured out where his meals come from, the udder should not look full to bursting, as it may have prior to foaling.

A telltale sign that the foal is not nursing normally is an udder that appears overly full or drops of milk that appear regularly on the teats. Alert your vet: these may be signs that your foal isn't feeling well.

Administering an Enema

A phosphate enema is recommended; you can use any brand from the drugstore that is safe for babies or children. Follow the directions on the box and never use force when giving an enema.

You may not need it, but it's wise to have another enema on hand, just in case. If you don't have an enema, mix 2 ounces of warm water with 1 to 3 teaspoons of mild dish soap. Warm it slightly; make sure it's not too hot. Put the mixture in an enema bottle or bag and administer.

Passing the Meconium

The meconium, the foal's first bowel movement, is dark, sticky, and fairly hard. The foal should pass the meconium within three hours after birth. Foals that pass the meconium shortly after birth will be hungry and continue nursing. This, in turn, causes the rest of the meconium to pass. Veterinarians often find that if the foal has an impacted meconium, the mare also has a retained placenta.

Many equine veterinarians recommend a single phosphate enema as part of the regular postfoaling routine. An enema will stimulate bowel function and help the foal pass the meconium quickly. This can be done before the foal gets to his feet for the first time, or just after nursing.

After he has passed the meconium, the new foal's bowel movements will be pasty and yellowish orange. Continue to keep an eye on him to make sure he is passing manure regularly. This is a simple matter if he is in a stall or small area; it is more difficult to observe once he and his mother are turned outside. After the foal has passed the meconium, you can safely assume he is passing manure normally, unless he exhibits any of the following signs:

- Holding up the tail in an arched manner ("squirrel tail")
- Abdominal straining, sometimes to the point of causing bleeding from the navel stump
- Rolling on his back with his head and neck outstretched

Urinating

Observe your new foal carefully to be sure he is urinating normally. Newborns will urinate frequently and in small quantities. The urine should be watery and clear. If there is any sign of discomfort or straining, particularly if no urine is released, contact the veterinarian.

It's not uncommon for urine to leak from the navel stump. Normally, when the umbilical cord breaks, a tubular structure inside the cord called the **urachus** should close naturally. If the urachus doesn't seal off, urine will trickle from the foal's navel stump.

Because the damp urine creates an ideal environment for bacterial growth and infection, your veterinarian will want to examine this condition promptly and treat it with medication if necessary. Re-treating the navel stump with iodine or Nolvasan is appropriate if the stump looks wet.

What to Watch for in the First 24 Hours and Shortly Thereafter

Pay close attention to your foal's attitude and physical condition, and call the vet if you notice anything out of the ordinary. Some potentially serious conditions can arise in the first few days, and prompt treatment can make a big difference in the final outcome.

Observe Foal Behavior

Take the foal's temperature within the first few hours after birth so you will have a baseline. Be aware, however, that because the foal's temperature alone is not the most reliable vital sign, it is crucial to observe the foal's behavior routinely. He should be nursing regularly, following the mare around the stall, and not exhibiting signs of straining or abdominal discomfort.

Signs of Septicemia

Septicemia is one of the leading causes of death among young foals and occurs when infection, which can be caused by a variety of organisms, enters the bloodstream and spreads rapidly, eventually affecting major organs.

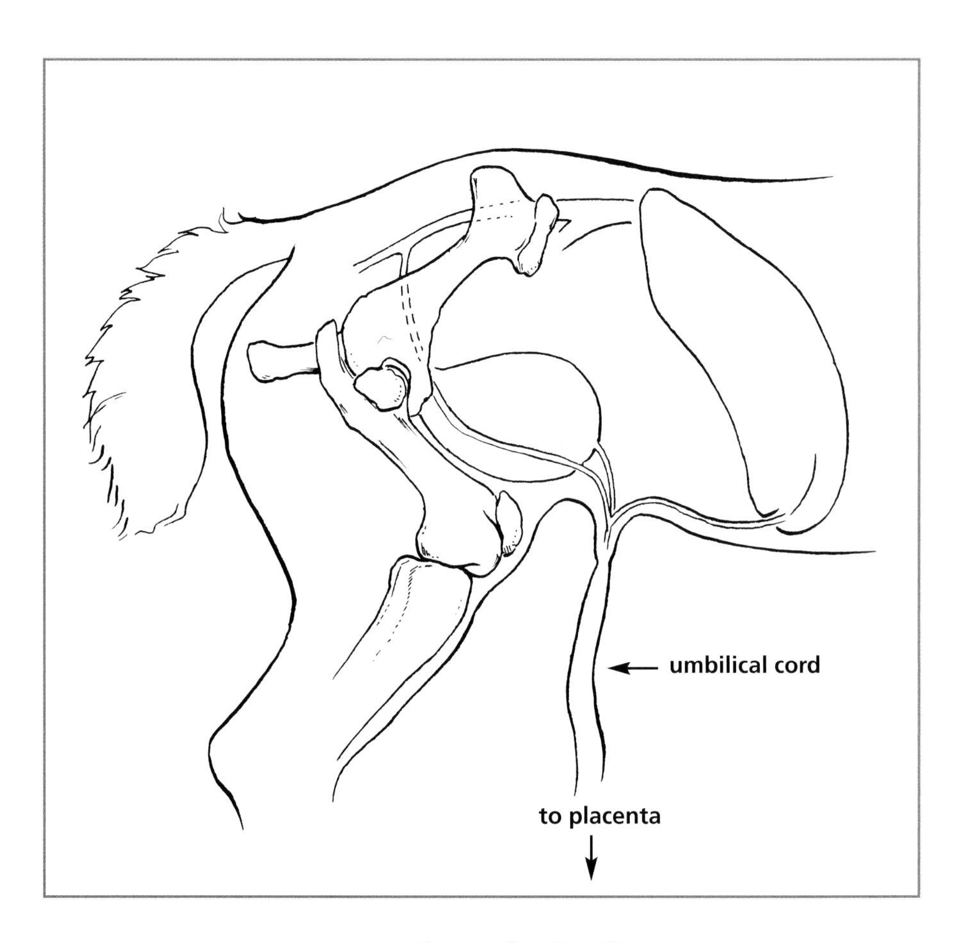

The foal's umbilical cord should break close to the abdomen. The cord contains the urachus as well as the umbilical arteries and vein.

Because most foals are exposed to potentially dangerous organisms soon after birth, the protection they receive from colostrum is a critical component in keeping them healthy. The risk of septicemia is why you must treat the navel stump as soon as the cord has broken and make sure the foaling area has been thoroughly cleaned and disinfected.

If you notice any of the following signs of septicemia, immediately alert your veterinarian. Prompt treatment with antibiotics and most likely intravenous fluids will be necessary.

- Loss of appetite
- Fever
- Bright green pupils in one or both eyes
- Change in respiration — either rapid or very slow
- Rapidly increasing depression, comalike state

Signs of Joint Ill

Joint ill is a common problem in foals that have had septicemia and can develop anytime from shortly after birth to three months of age. The first symptom of joint ill is lameness, as the affected joints become swollen, hot, and painful. Because permanent damage to the joints and bones can occur, prompt treatment is necessary.

Lameness in newborn and young foals is usually a significant clinical sign and should be investigated and treated without delay. Better to treat any sign of lameness as if it were a joint-ill episode until proved otherwise.

A lengthy course of antibiotic treatment is required when a foal is diagnosed with joint ill. The vet may need to flush joint cavities to remove harmful enzymes, and inject antibiotics directly into the joint capsules.

If you notice any of the following symptoms of joint ill, notify the vet right away:

- Lameness
- Hot, swollen joints
- Fever
- Foal stops nursing and becomes lethargic

Your Mare after Foaling

Your mare should normally pass the placenta, or afterbirth, within an hour after foaling. If she has not passed it within three hours, contact the vet.

Once she has passed the placenta and her foal has nursed, you can feed the mare a warm wheat bran mash. Or give her half of her normal feed ration and wet it down with warm water until it is "sloppy." Either way, this should be her first meal after she has presented you with a brand-new foal. Because the bran mash is a significant change in diet from her normal ration, ask your vet if she recommends the mash or just wetting down the regular feed.

Offering warm, wet feed is both "comfort food" for the mare and a way to rehydrate her. Adding molasses to the mash or feed will also make her want to drink more water. If her manure is hard and dry, which can happen if she is not eating fresh grass or drinking enough water, the vet may advise you to feed her more than one mash over the next couple of days, or to continue wetting down her feed for a few days.

Note: For many years, horse owners believed that bran mash worked as a laxative and helped remove sand from the intestine. Although this has been proved false, a warm bran mash is tasty and appreciated by most horses from time to time. *Caution!* Because wheat bran has a high phosphorus content, it shouldn't typically be fed more than once or twice a week. Also, avoid feeding it to horses under the age of three, as too much phosphorus can cause bone development problems.

Taking Temperature

1. To take the foal's temperature, lubricate a digital rectal thermometer with the lubricant in your foaling kit or with petroleum jelly.
2. Have someone hold the foal so he doesn't struggle.
3. Lift the foal's tail and insert the lubricated end of the thermometer into the anus.
4. Hold the thermometer in place for at least 10 seconds, or until it signals that enough time has passed for an accurate reading. Don't leave the thermometer unattended!

The average normal foal temperature is 99° to 102°F.

First Vet Visit, Day One

Your veterinarian should examine the foal the day it is born to determine if it appears healthy and if there are any deviations from normal. She will use a stethoscope to listen to the foal's heart and lungs, and will examine the umbilical area to be sure the navel stump has been treated properly and looks normal. She will also check to see if the foal has any damage from the birth process, such as broken ribs, bruises, any redness or hemorrhage in the sclera of the eyes, or discolored pupils. Because newborn foals are fragile, this first-day exam is a smart move to establish good health.

Making Your Own Wheat Bran Mash

3 pounds wheat bran
1 cup dark blackstrap molasses
Approximately 4 cups hot water (more if the mare likes it "sloppy")
Handful of grain

Mix all the ingredients together and allow to cool slightly. The mash should be warm, not hot.

Blood Tests for the Foal

If the mare didn't leak much colostrum before delivery and the foal has nursed well shortly after birth, chances are good that he will be fine. But you should still request an **IgG test** (immunoglobulin G test, also known as **failure of passive transfer** test), which will show if the foal has absorbed enough antibodies from the colostrum. This simple test, which is typically performed 18 to 24 hours after birth, can be very important to your foal's future and gives your vet a head start on preventing problems. Diarrhea, pneumonia, and joint ill are some common problems in foals with low levels of antibodies.

The vet will draw a small amount of blood from the foal for the IgG test. The blood is sent to a lab or clinic for testing and the results will indicate if the antibody levels are adequate, if

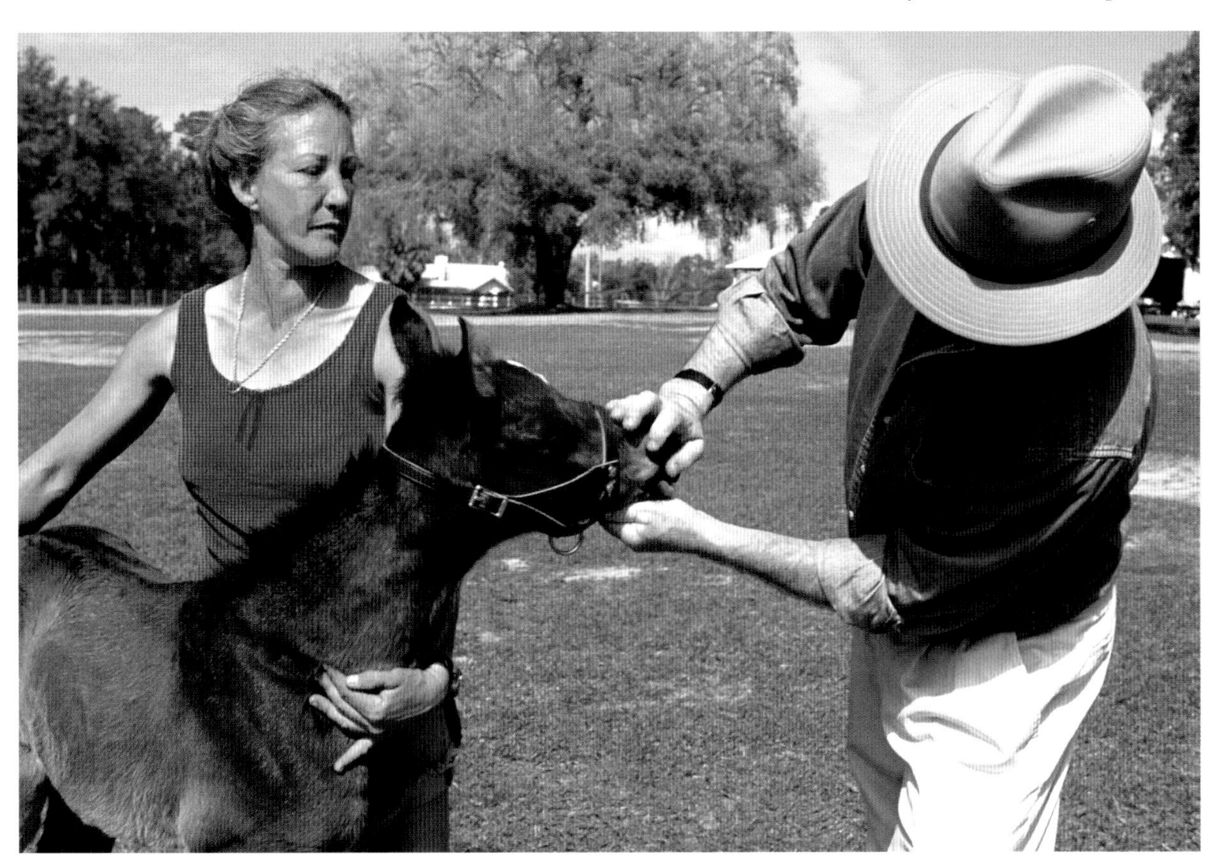

A physical exam by your veterinarian is standard on the foal's first day.

there are deficiencies in the colostrum, or if the foal is having trouble absorbing the milk.

If test results reveal low levels of antibodies, the vet will likely give the foal a transfusion of **plasma,** which is unclotted blood with the red cells removed. She will order this plasma from a biological supply company that maintains herds of properly vaccinated horses that have tested negative for contagious equine diseases. Plasma is collected from these horses and either frozen or freeze-dried. Because the plasma comes from donor horses that have been extensively vaccinated, the transfusion will transfer protection to the new foal.

Once it arrives, the vet thaws the plasma, warms it, and administers it intravenously to

Watch the Mare!

Mares become quite protective of their new babies. Always move around a new mom with caution and pay close attention to her body language. If her ears go back, she is telling you to watch out! Have someone available to hold the mare whenever you must handle the foal.

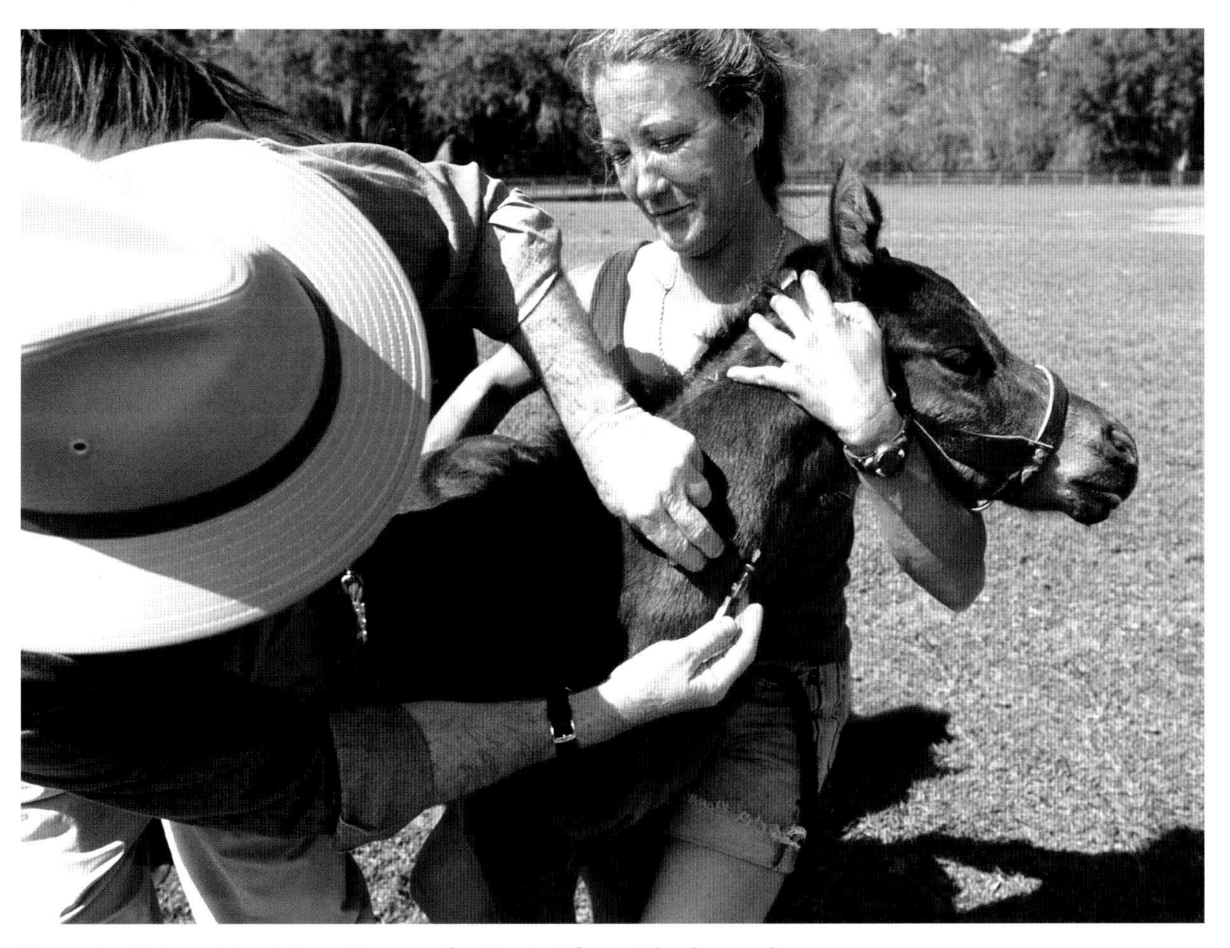

The vet will draw blood from the new foal to test for antibodies and to ensure that the blood count is normal.

the foal. Usually the vet will sedate the foal to keep him still during this process.

The vet may also want to draw blood to run a **CBC** (complete blood count) on your foal from 12 to 24 hours after birth. If the CBC comes back with abnormal results, the foal may need to receive antibiotics for a few days.

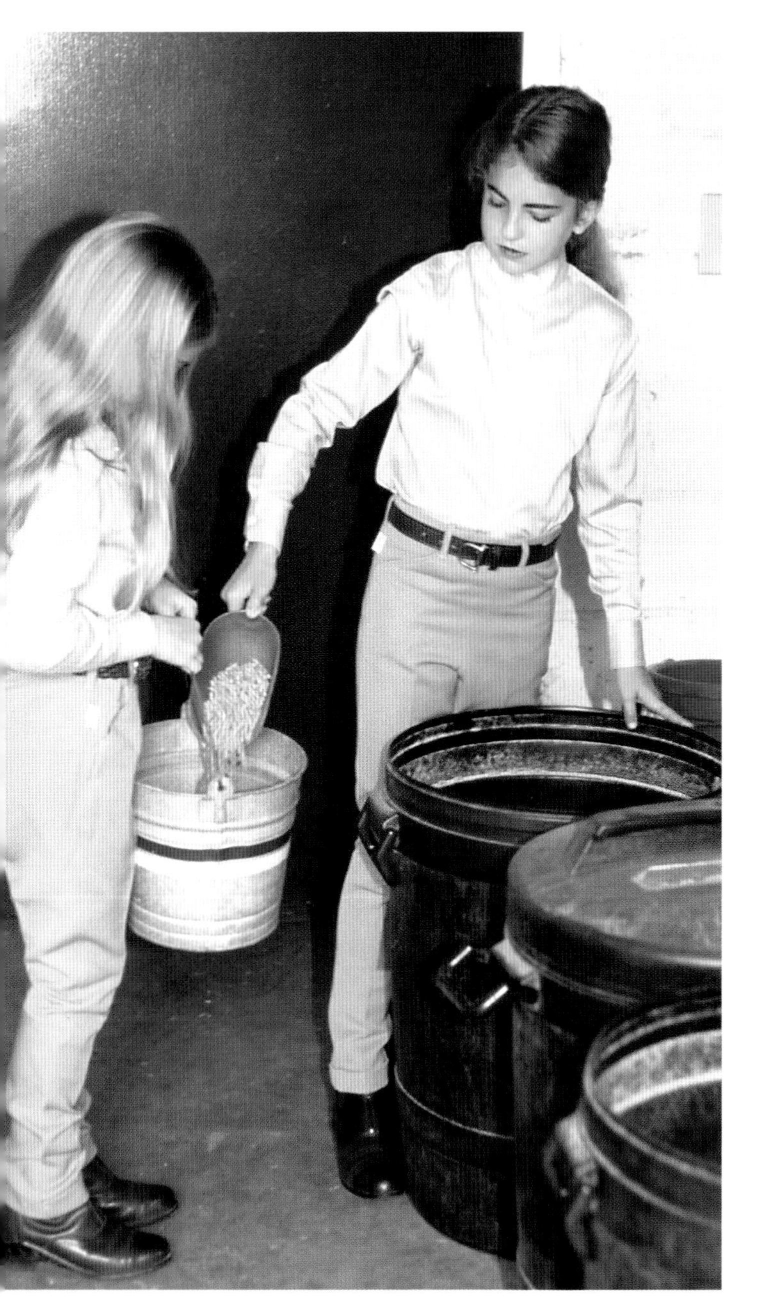

On some farms, it is common to put newborn foals on antibiotics for the first 72 hours after birth just as a precaution, even if the foals appear normal and healthy. Discuss this with your veterinarian before your mare foals so you know what the plan is. This short treatment can be helpful in preventing septicemia (see page 41), but unless the foal is actually ill, avoid longer treatment because it may produce resistance to antibiotics.

Vet Check for the Mare

Your vet will probably give the mare a brief postfoaling exam on the day after to check if she injured any tissues during delivery.

This is a good time to ask about changes in the mare's feed routine. Your vet may tell you to give the mare her regular feed after the first bran mash or recommend wetting her regular feed for the next few days after foaling.

The mare needs quality feed with adequate protein to help her body produce milk. Good leafy legume hay, such as alfalfa or an alfalfa mix, is recommended for most lactating mares, along with a balanced commercial feed designed especially for lactating mares. Avoid abrupt changes in feed or feeding routine, particularly after the stress of foaling. If the vet suggests any changes, incorporate them gradually over the course of a week or so.

Always be sure your mare has plenty of fresh water and trace mineral salt available free choice.

Watch for Dehydration

Sometimes a mare won't drink as much water as usual just before and right after the stressful demands of foaling. Do the "pinch test" on the mare in the days after foaling or any time you

The mare needs quality feed to maintain her own body condition *and* produce milk for the new foal.

have concerns about dehydration. Pinch the skin in the middle of the horse's neck and pull it slightly away from the body. In a healthy, hydrated horse, as soon as you let go the skin should flatten. If it stays "tented" or pinched at all, the horse is already dehydrated.

The great majority of horses love the sweet taste of molasses, which also encourages them to drink water. You can offer a small amount of straight dark blackstrap molasses in a pan for the mare to lick, or flavor a 5-gallon bucket of water by adding a half cup or so of molasses directly to it. If you hang two buckets of water in the stall, one unflavored and one containing the molasses, many horses prefer the molasses water and will drink it first. This is a simple and effective way to encourage horses to drink.

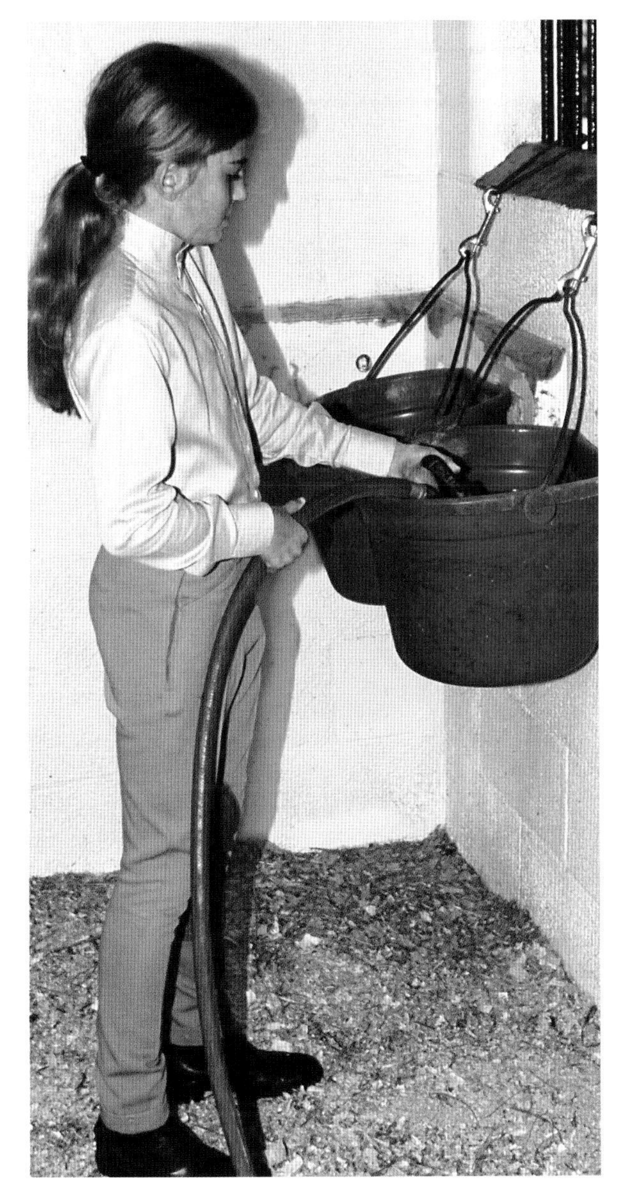

Plenty of fresh water is a must for the mare. Keep an eye on her bucket to make sure she is drinking normally.

Postfoaling "Blues"

If your mare looks and acts tired on the day of giving birth, she probably is — and with good reason. Delivering a foal is hard work, and is tougher on some mares than on others, especially if she is in her teens or older or has had many foals.

After foaling, the mare typically has sore abdominal muscles, and if she hasn't been drinking and eating normally, her digestive system may not be functioning fully. She may act lethargic or depressed or not be as active as usual. Keep an eye on her to be sure she is passing manure regularly. Some postfoaling mares just need to rest and be pampered a bit. Other mares benefit from veterinary treatment. If your mare isn't acting herself or seems uncomfortable, consult your veterinarian.

Getting Outside

Fresh air, sunshine, and a little time spent outdoors on the first day will be good for both mother and baby, provided the foal is strong and healthy and the weather is mild. Turn them out in a small area and just by themselves at first. Don't put them next to any other horses — they may threaten the baby, even over a fence.

The best situation is a small corral with safe fencing that opens directly out of the stall. This way the mare can move around more than she would in the confines of a stall, but not so much as to tire the newborn. You absolutely do

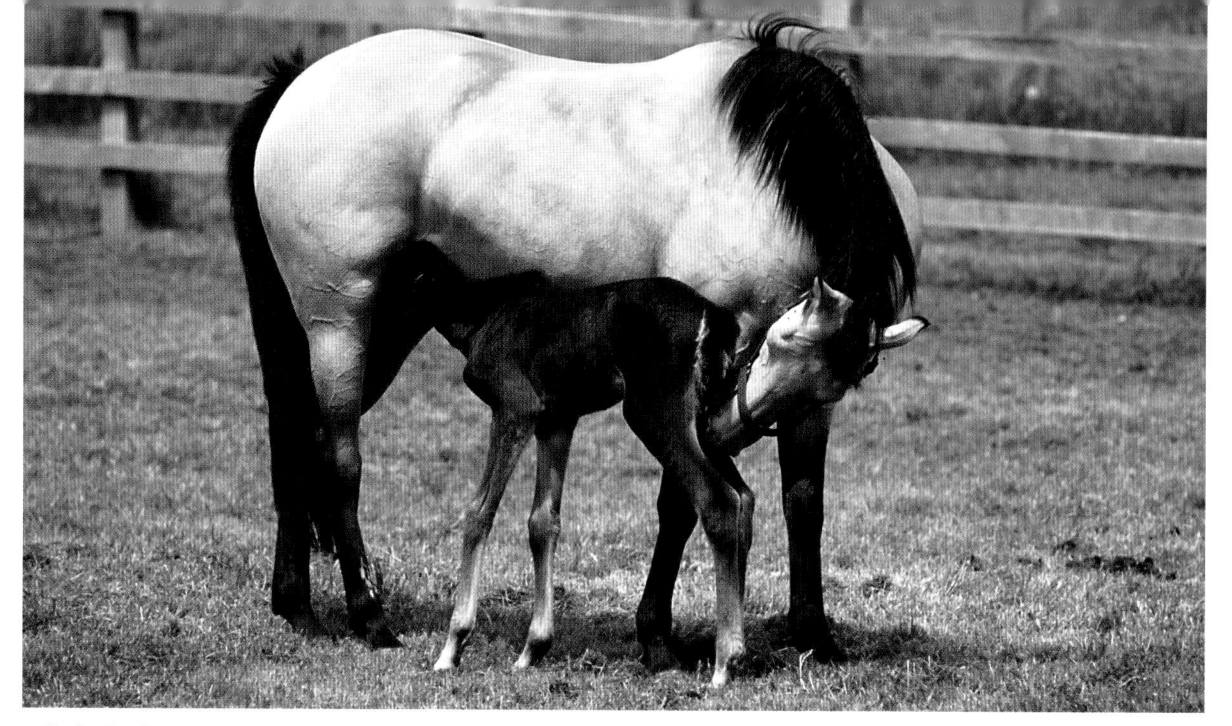

A little fresh air on the first day is good for both mare and foal, provided the weather is mild.

not want to create a dangerous situation in which the mare runs in a large area and her new foal tries to keep up, which can severely exhaust and stress him. If the mare is too active, put her and the foal back inside the stall.

If your foal has weak legs or any kind of angular limb problems, the vet will probably recommend that mare and foal stay in the stall for a few days, until the foal is stronger.

You should have one other person — preferably two others — on hand for turning out mare and foal the first time. One person leads the mare while the other guides the foal, one arm cradling it around the chest and the other arm around its hindquarters. A third person can help open and close gates. *Don't, under any circumstances, try to lead the newborn foal by a halter or lead rope! It's too soon.*

First lead the mare through the gate and then turn her around so she is facing her baby and the person holding it. Don't release the foal until the mare is facing it. There have been unfortunate incidents in which an excited mare kicks out when turned loose and accidentally strikes and injures her foal.

Dealing with Tragedy

The great majority of mares foal without much difficulty. Unfortunately, however, there are times when a foal dies during or shortly after birth, and occasions when the mare dies.

If the foal is born dead or dies at birth, don't immediately remove the body from the stall. The mare needs to accept her foal has died. If the body is removed before she has come to this realization, she may become frantic. Leave the body in the stall until she no longer acts interested. This may take less than an hour, but it can take longer, depending on the mare. She will sniff and probably lick the dead foal, but will soon come to accept the fact that her foal is gone. Then you can remove the body.

Because the mare will have a full udder, talk with the vet about what to feed her, how to reduce her milk production, and how to "dry" her up. The vet or another horseman in the area may know of an orphan foal in need of a mother, in which case you may be able to relieve your mare's distress and help another foal whose mother has died.

Raising an Orphan

When the mare dies during or shortly after foaling, the best scenario is to find a surrogate mother to raise the foal. In some areas with a large breeding farm population, there are people who have available **nurse mares.** These are mares bred to have a foal each year so they are on call in case a mare dies and her foal needs a surrogate mother.

When this happens, the nurse mare's own foal is raised on a bucket or bottle and the nurse mare is transported to the farm of the orphan foal, where she raises that baby as her own. The owner of the foal is responsible for the care, feeding, and maintenance of the nurse mare until the foal is weaned, and typically pays a fee to the owner of the nurse mare. The nurse mare is usually bred again so that she will deliver another foal the following year.

Raising a Foal by Hand

If a nurse mare or surrogate is not available, you can raise an orphan foal by hand. This is a challenging task, but certainly possible. Quality mare's milk replacers, such as Foal-Lac, are sold through feed stores. Alternatively, you can make your own formula using goat's milk or 2 percent cow's milk to which you add a small amount of honey or corn syrup to increase the carbohydrates. If you make your own formula, the vet will prescribe the proper ratios.

The first days and weeks of life are critical, as the foal needs to nurse at least every hour for his first several days, and only slightly less frequently for the next few weeks. If he did not receive colostrum from his mother, he must receive a colostrum supplement. It is always best to obtain actual colostrum instead of a supplement. Ask your vet if there are local farms that maintain a colostrum bank. Some farms with multiple mares will collect and freeze colostrum for just such emergency situations.

After the orphan foal has received the colostrum or colostrum supplement, bottle-feed him every half hour to an hour for the first five days (see page 39). Use a regular plastic baby bottle with the nipple hole slightly enlarged. Offer about eight ounces at a time; newborn foals typically nurse frequently and drink small amounts. This amount can be increased to 16 ounces per feeding for the first seven to ten days if the foal will drink it.

After this point, you can usually feed the foal once an hour during the day but just every couple of hours at night. The amount of milk should increase as the time between feedings

How Foals Compare with Other Infants

Foals are among several precocial species that are active and walking, even running, within a very short time after birth. Take a look at how they compare to some other newborns. Shown is the approximate amount of time required for the new baby to stand and walk on his own.

Foal — 1 to 2 hours
Calf — 1 to 2 hours
Lamb/kid — 1 to 2 hours
Puppy — 3 weeks (crawls prior to walking)
Tiger cub — 2 to 3 weeks (crawls prior to walking)
Chimpanzee — able to walk at 6 months, but likes to ride on mom's back for at least 2 years
Human baby — 9 to 13 months (crawls prior to walking)

increases. For example, if you are feeding 16 ounces every hour and the foal is drinking it all, offer 24 to 32 ounces if you spread out the feedings to every two hours. Eventually, you can switch the foal from a bottle to drinking milk out of a small bucket.

When raising an orphan, you must be in regular contact with your vet, who will advise you on adjusting the amount of milk and the feeding schedule according to the needs of the individual foal. She will also tell you when to introduce solid feed (usually within the first month), which will cut down on the amount of milk replacer needed until the foal can be safely weaned. A common problem with orphans is that they develop scours (diarrhea), so keep an eye out for this and consult the vet if it continues.

Reinforce good manners whenever you are handling the orphan foal. Because they are hand-fed, orphans may become spoiled or even dangerous, so it is important that your foal respect you.

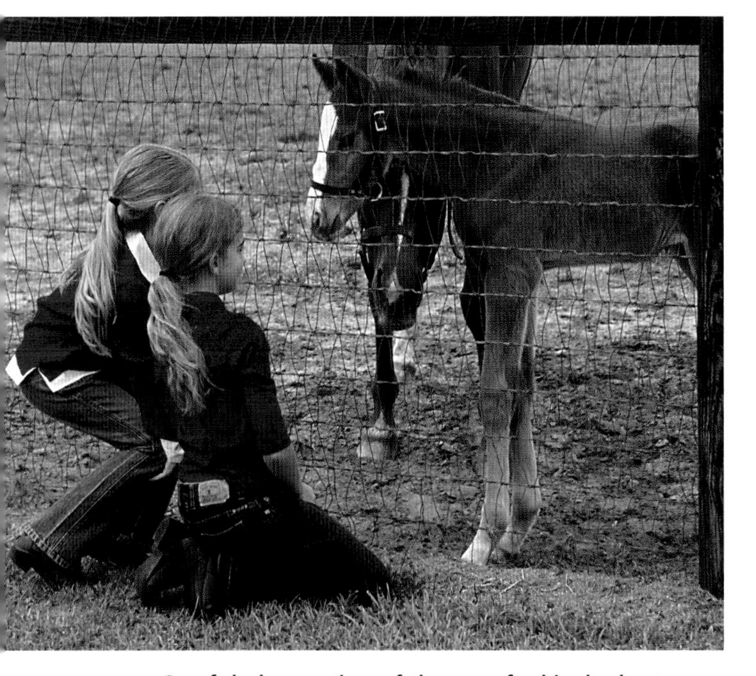

Careful observation of the new foal is the best way to detect anything out of the ordinary.

First-Day Checklist

Within 2 Hours

- ☐ Treat foal's navel with iodine or Nolvasan immediately after cord breaks
- ☐ Clean mare's udder and hindquarters before foal nurses for first time
- ☐ Foal must receive colostrum as soon as possible after birth
- ☐ Make sure foal is nursing well
- ☐ Give enema to foal
- ☐ Mare expels placenta
- ☐ Examine placenta to be sure it's intact
- ☐ Give bran mash or wet feed to mare
- ☐ Have fresh water and hay available for mare at all times
- ☐ Clean up foaling stall and add fresh bedding

Within 3 to 4 Hours

- ☐ Make sure mare is passing manure
- ☐ Foal should pass meconium

Within 12 Hours

- ☐ Watch to see that foal is urinating and passing manure normally
- ☐ Deworm mare with ivermectin product
- ☐ Postfoaling exam for foal and mare
- ☐ Blood drawn from foal 12 to 24 hours after birth for testing
- ☐ Short time outdoors in small, safe area, unless vet says otherwise

WHAT'S NORMAL, WHAT'S NOT: The Newborn Foal

Normal:

- Temperature 99° to 102°F
- Alert and aware of surroundings
- Bonding with dam
- Frequent vigorous nursing
- Frequent short naps
- Passing thick, dark, sticky meconium (first bowel movement) within first few hours
- Clear, watery urine

Not Normal:

- Elevated or below-normal temperature
- Dull, lethargic attitude
- Nursing infrequently
- Sleeping for long periods
- Holding the tail elevated and arched
- Rolling on back with head and neck outstretched
- Straining when trying to urinate or move bowels
- Urine or blood dripping from navel stump

WHAT'S NORMAL, WHAT'S NOT: The New Mother

Normal:

- Temperature 99°F to 101.5°F
- May act tired, but shouldn't appear dull or "spacey"
- Concern for foal, may include vigorous licking and sniffing
- Protective attitude toward newborn
- Average to hearty appetite

Not Normal:

- Elevated or below-normal temperature
- Dull, lethargic attitude
- Lack of interest or little interest in foal
- Violent or aggressive behavior toward foal
- No appetite
- Lying down for long periods
- Continued pawing (once labor is over)
- Sweating (once labor is over)
- Continued straining

5

Handling during the First Days and Weeks

Unlike humans, puppies, and kittens, the foal is capable of learning at a very young age. His mind files away his earliest experiences and he never forgets them. Thus, it is important that your first interactions with the foal are positive ones.

With proper handling, a newborn foal will develop into a trusting and respectful adult horse. Handling him the right way in the first days and weeks can reduce the likelihood of future injuries to both horse and human. It will teach him to be respectful, less afraid, gentle, and cooperative. A big advantage to working with a foal is that you are starting with a clean slate and don't have to correct any previous learning problems.

Early Handling Makes a Difference

Not so many years ago, even experienced horsemen and -women thought it foolhardy to spend much time handling young foals. The standard practice was to intervene only if there was trouble and to leave the rest to nature. A foal would be caught for veterinary or blacksmith visits, but otherwise he was simply left to run at his mother's side until it was time for weaning. After weaning, foals ran in a herd with other young horses, and as a result experienced very little consistent handling until they were broken and trained to ride.

Indeed, the new foal needs time to bond with his dam and to settle into his new world. However, you can interact with him a great deal during those first days and weeks, setting the stage for a good partnership.

Bonding with the Dam

In the wild, it is critical that the newborn foal bond quickly with his mother. Because the horse's main survival behavior is to run from danger, his instinct to stay close to and follow his mother immediately may mean the difference between life and death.

Our domesticated horses aren't usually placed in situations where they have to flee to survive. But a foal will still instinctively bond with his mother right after birth, soon learning that his mother is the source of food, protection, and companionship.

Horses are herd animals and there is always a leader (or **alpha horse**) in the group. The others respect and depend on this dominant horse to find watering spots and good grazing and to keep them from danger. A foal that is properly handled when very young learns that the human is the alpha figure, and that he can be trusting and submissive to that human without cause for fear.

Bonding with Humans

On the day of his birth, you will already have handled the foal to dip his navel, administer an enema, try on the halter, and hold him for the first vet visit. Now expand on your initial contact by spending daily time with the mare and foal. In the early days and weeks, make it a

The foal will instinctively bond with his mother right after birth.

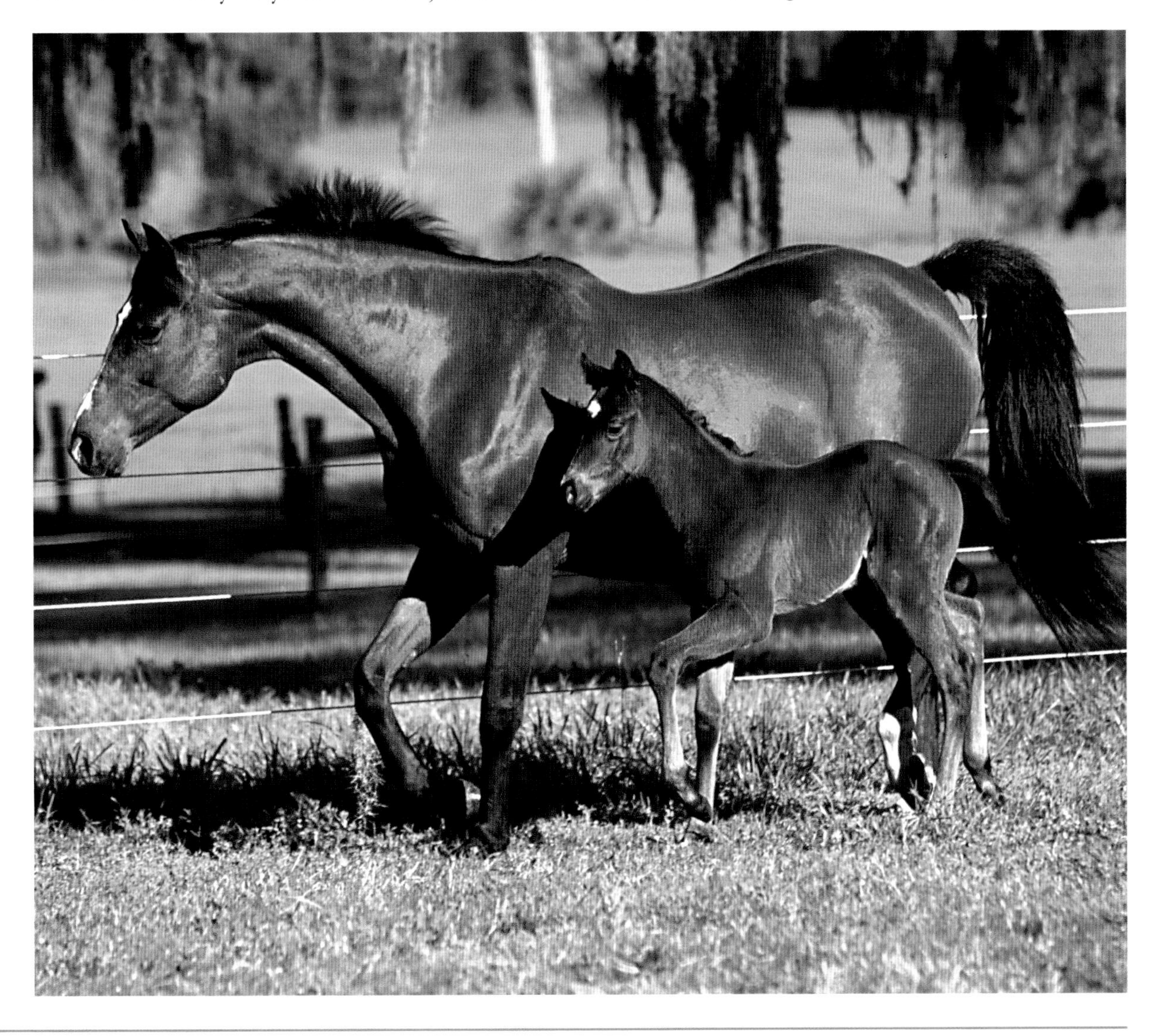

habit to touch the foal often every day. When you take the mare and foal in and out of the stall, take advantage of this opportunity to rub and touch the foal all over his body.

How to Handle a Foal

Most people want to pat a horse, but this is not how horses touch each other. Rub or stroke your foal instead of patting. Start rubbing his shoulder, not his face or nose. Once the foal is comfortable with having his shoulder rubbed, move up to his withers, then along his neck to his head. Rub along the foal's back and rump, and run your hands up and down his legs. It's simple to teach the young foal to let you pick up his feet if you start at an early age.

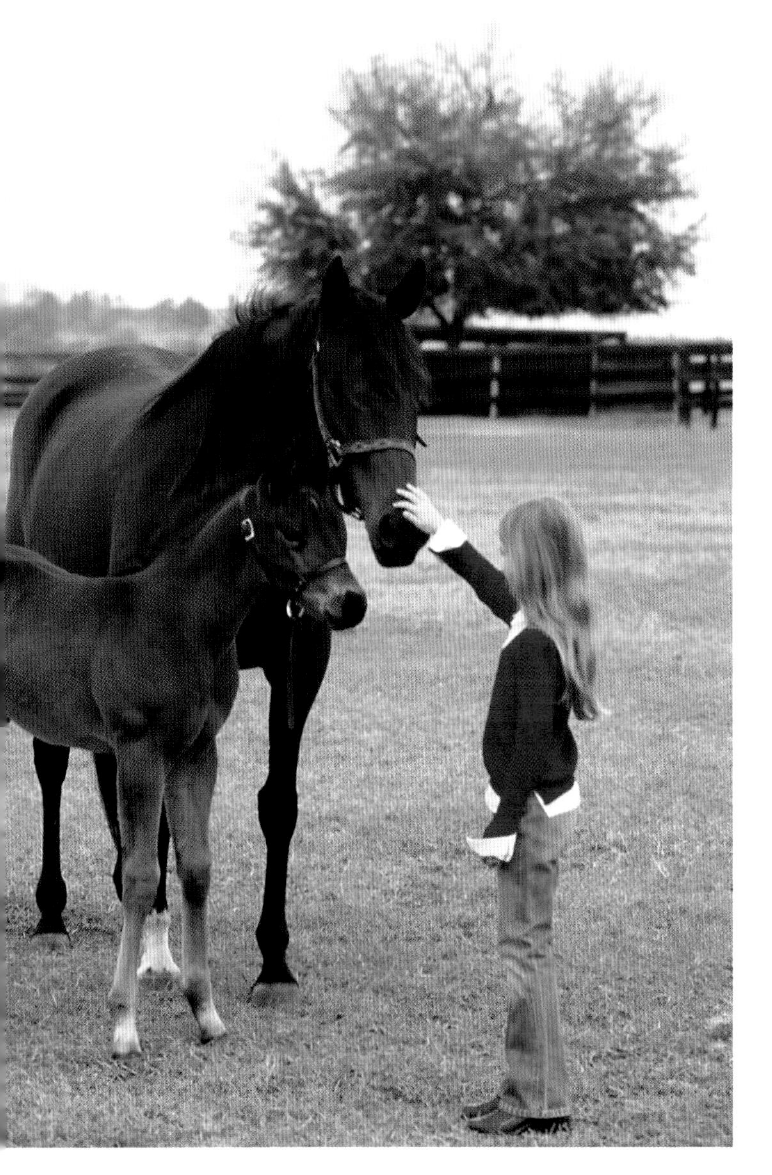

Use a light touch when stroking a horse's face.

Precautions: Safety First!

Take into consideration your mare's temperament and background when handling the young foal. If you have a nervous, young, or overly protective mare, her attitude may interfere with your early handling of the foal. More important, she can be dangerous for you to work around.

Many mares will ease up after the first few days of motherhood, once they realize you are not going to hurt the baby. Even if you have a relaxed, quiet mare, however, someone else should be present to halter and hold her whenever you are working with the foal. Safety must always be your first goal.

Keep in mind that if you have an ill-mannered, unschooled mare, it is unrealistic to expect her foal to be unflappable and easygoing. The foal learns and inherits much of his behavior from his dam, which is why you should think twice about breeding a mare with a nasty disposition. Yes, you can try to shape the foal's nature by spending time working with him, but the majority of those first important months will be spent in his mother's company. He will have a tendency to mimic her behavior, good or bad.

You can, and should, vary the pressure of your touch, depending on where you are stroking the foal. Most foals love to be vigorously scratched or rubbed at their withers, but use a lighter touch on the face, legs, and sensitive areas.

Handling his entire head, especially his ears, at an early age can help prevent head-shyness when the horse is older. The foal quickly learns that he has nothing to fear from submitting to your touch.

Avoid "Horseplay"

It can be tempting to engage in "horseplay" with the young foal, but it is never a wise decision to chase and run with him as though you were another horse. The foal needs to think of you as a leader, not as his buddy or equal. Many people have made the mistake of letting a foal push them around or chase them in the field, thinking this is cute and that he will outgrow this behavior. Others teach their foal to rear up on command, unaware of how dangerous this "trick" will be once the horse is fully grown.

What the foal learns now, he will remember. If he can climb all over you as a baby, he won't have any reason to think this is wrong when he is a big strong yearling. If you teach him to rear up and put his front feet on your shoulders as a foal, he won't understand why you're disciplining him for trying to do this when he's older.

Leave horseplay to the horses. You will have plenty of time to interact with your foal and make a positive impression without sending him mixed messages.

You're the Boss

Although the foal should let you rub and touch him, don't make the mistake of letting *him* rub on *you.* Horses rub on each other, but you are not a horse. If you let the foal start pushing against you or rubbing on you when you handle him, he is not showing respect. He is thinking of you as a peer, not as a leader.

Regular handling during the first few days has made this foal comfortable with being touched all over.

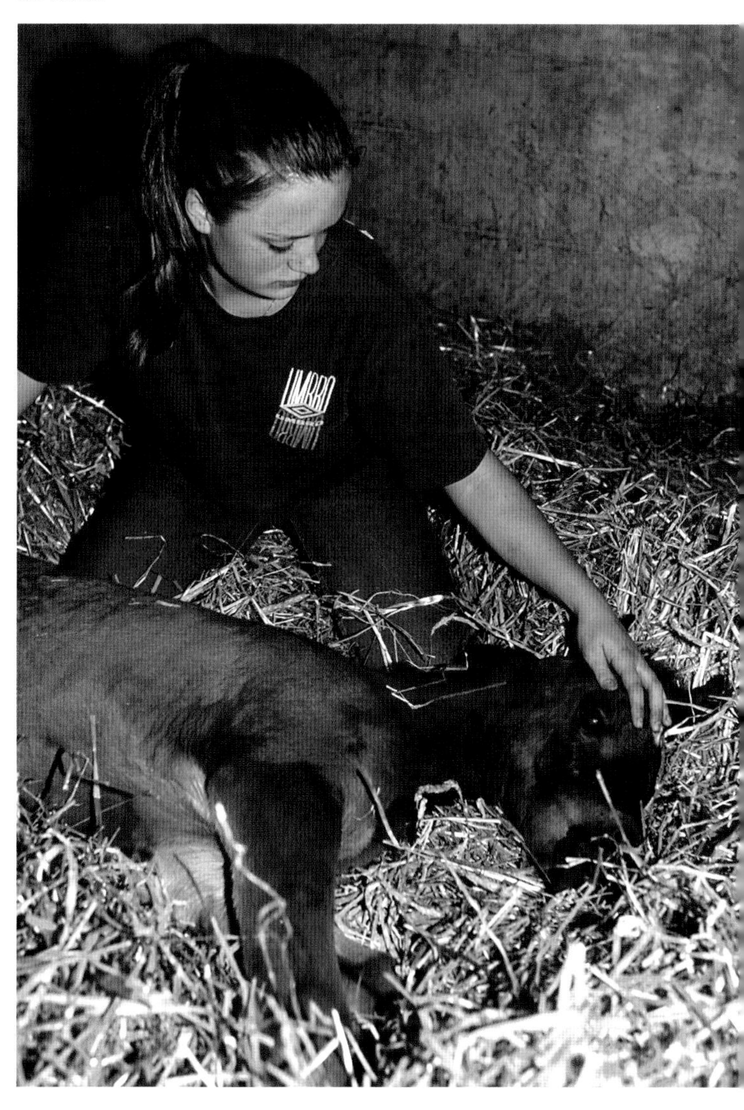

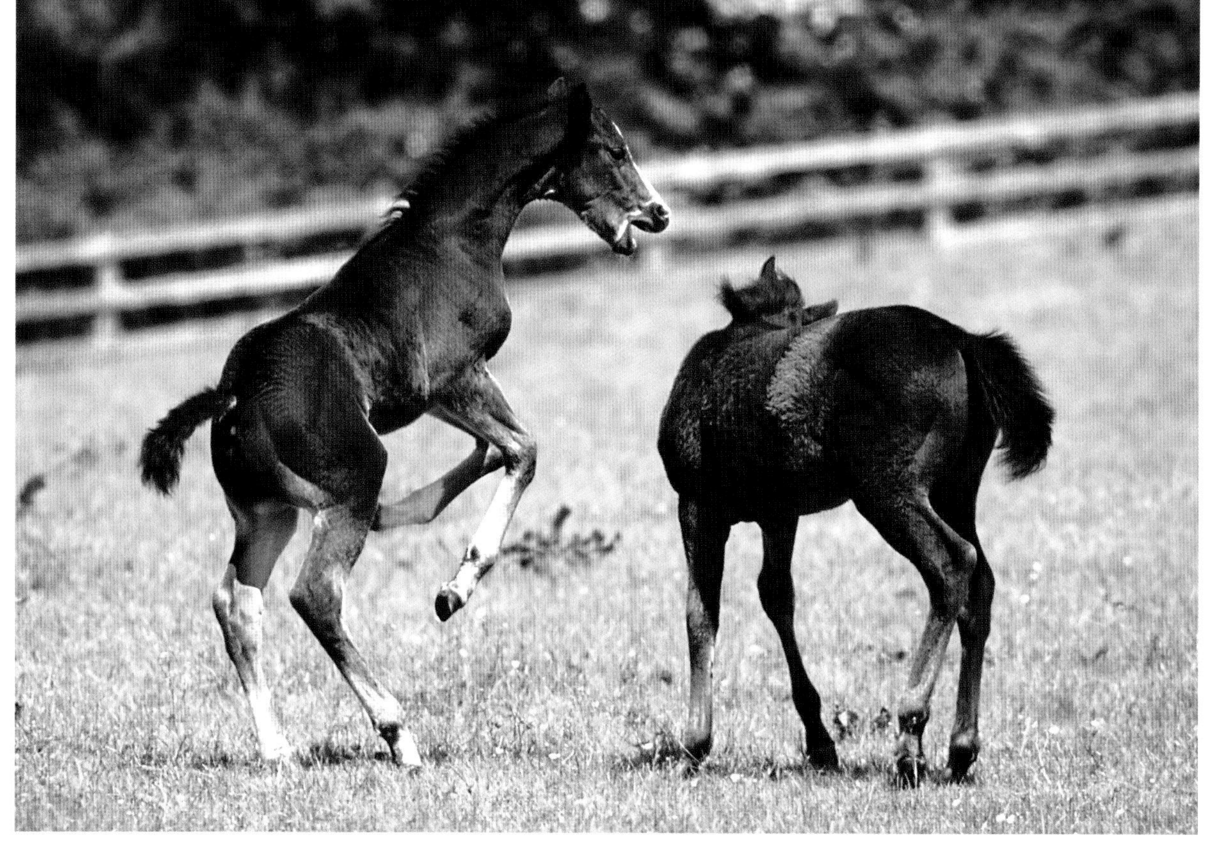

Leave horseplay to the horses. Never play with your horse as if you were another foal.

Restraining the Young Foal

A young or small foal can be easily restrained or held by cradling him. Standing to the side of the foal, place one arm around his chest, just below the neck. Your other arm should be around his hindquarters, resting below his tail. This way you can guide him forward or hold him in place. The newborn foal should be cradled in this way when led in and out of the stall until he learns to lead.

Use the least amount of restraint necessary so the foal does not struggle or sink to the ground. Think of your arms as a corral, using restraint only if he is trying to escape. When he relaxes, stop all pressure and restraint on his body.

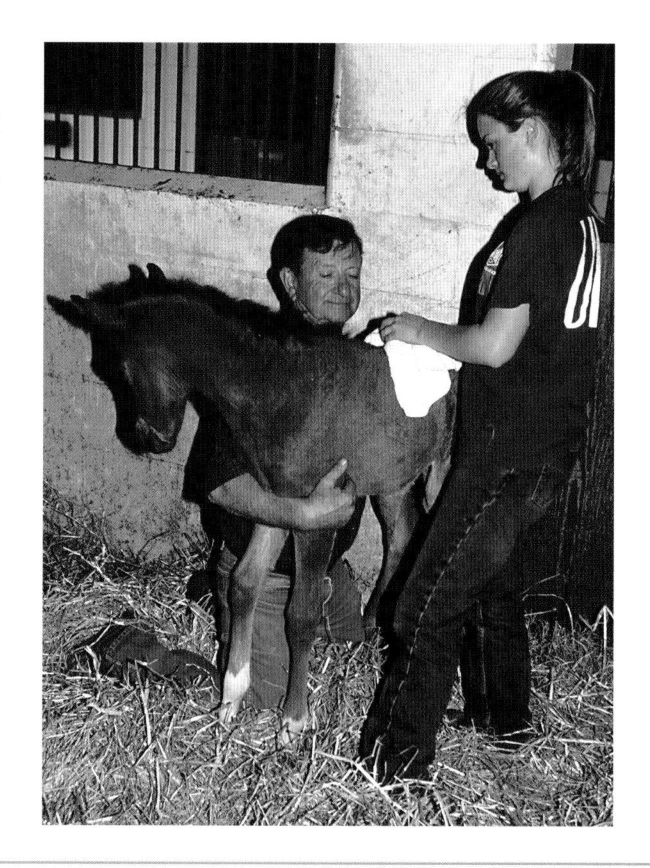

Comfortable being touched by human hands, this young foal is gently cradled while his owner rubs him with a grooming rag. Don't cradle the foal tightly, or he will struggle or sink to the ground.

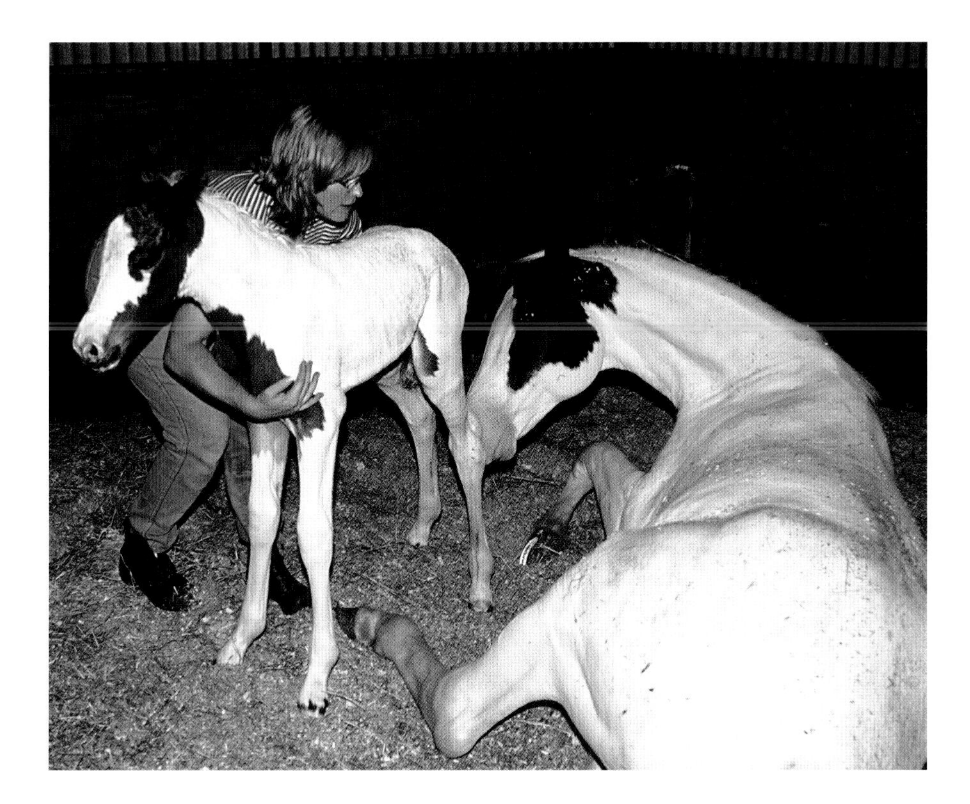

You can restrain the foal by cradling him with one arm around his chest and the other at his hindquarters.

Consistency Is Crucial

It is important to be consistent when handling a young foal. Much like a child, the foal will repeatedly test you to see just what you will let him get away with. He won't understand if you let him rub his head on you one day, but discipline him for doing this the next day. It's up to you to set boundaries and maintain them.

The foal has no problem with you being his leader, but that doesn't mean he won't routinely try to see if you are indeed still "the boss." Horses do this within the herd all the time, since it is to their advantage to move up in the pecking order. By teaching the foal to accept your touch, you are replacing his fear of humans with trust. Respect is developed as the foal learns not to violate your space and realizes that you, as the alpha figure, can control his movements.

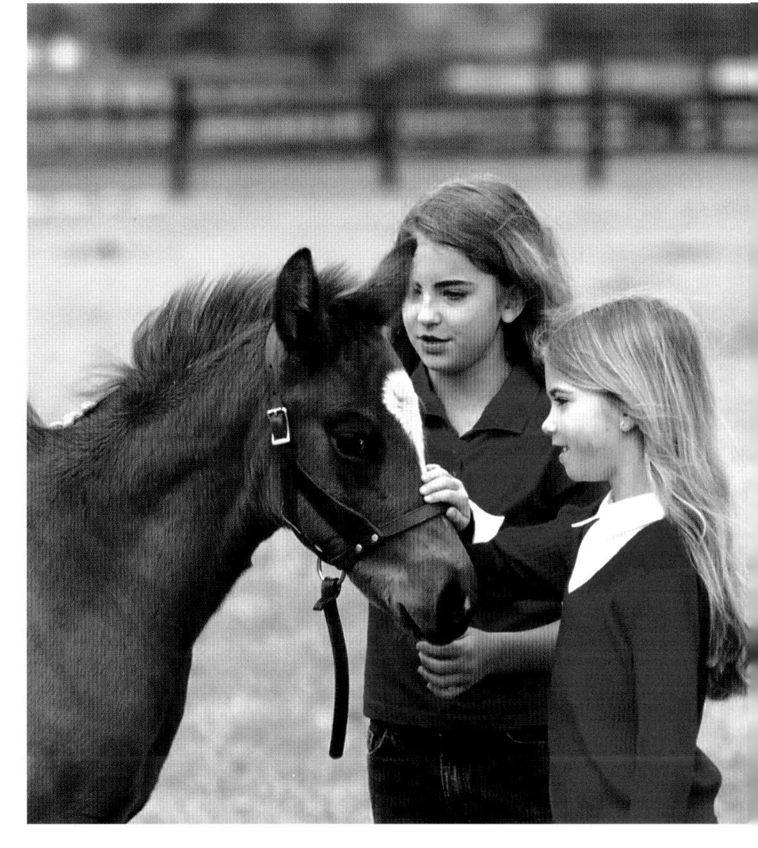

To avoid turning into a spoiled foal, he must respect you and not think of you as his equal.

6

The First Weeks

During the first days and weeks of life, the foal's mind is a blank slate waiting to be filled. Make this a period of positive experiences and lessons, because what the foal learns now will stay with him for the rest of his life.

Haltering the Foal

Try to halter the foal on the first day. He will quickly get used to the halter if he wears it daily. Halter the mare and foal only when you are handling and leading them; remove the halters whenever they are in their stall or turned out. This leaves no possibility of the horses catching or snagging the halter on anything.

Leather halters are always safer than nylon. Leather will usually break if stressed; nylon is so strong that even an adult horse may not be able to break it. If a horse catches a nylon halter on something, it's usually the horse or the object that breaks or gives, not the halter, and the results are often disastrous. You can always replace a broken halter.

Fitting the Halter

Your new foal will need several different halters as he grows. Start with a leather newborn halter designed to fit the foal at birth. The noseband has a figure-eight shape, so it doesn't rest low on the nose or face when properly adjusted. The strap that goes over the **poll,** just behind the foal's ears, should be adjustable on both sides. Adjust it so that the noseband doesn't hang down and the whole halter fits fairly snug. Too loose is too dangerous!

To check for proper adjustment, slide a finger under the noseband and straps all around the halter. If you can't do this readily, the halter is too tight. If you can slip several fingers under the straps and noseband, it's not snug enough.

If the halter is loose, the foal may catch it on something in the stall, such as a bucket, hook, or latch. Outside, a loose strap can snag on branches and bushes. A foal can even catch his own hoof in a too-loose halter when trying to scratch himself. It is up to you to imagine situations in which the foal can get in trouble and then make it impossible for those situations to occur. Forethought and common-sense horsemanship will eliminate many potential problems.

Don't forget to check the fit of the mare's halter, using the same guidelines to make sure it is neither too tight nor too loose. A foal will often sniff and paw at his mother when the mare lies down, so if her halter is loose, the foal could manage to get a hoof caught in her halter. This is another reason why the safest scenario is to remove their halters when mare and foal are loose.

Make sure to adjust the foal's halter properly so that it is neither too loose nor too snug. You can see the front part of the butt rope around this youngster's chest.

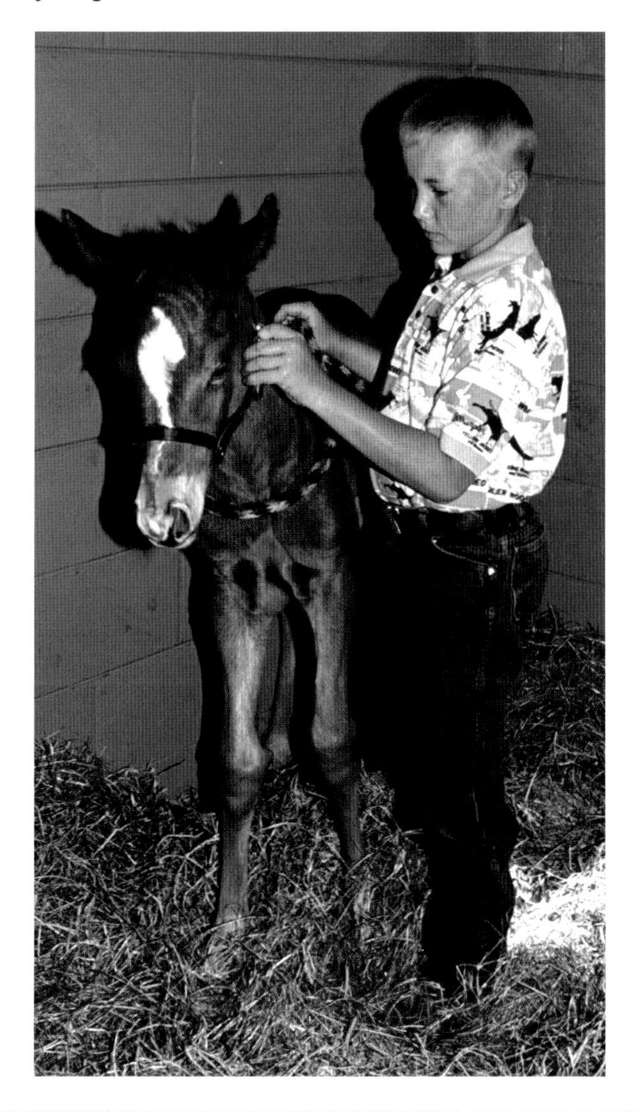

Handling the Haltered Foal

Some people worry that if they take off the halter, a horse will be difficult to catch. The fact is that it's not safe or sensible to have a horse you can catch only by grabbing at the halter. The more time you invest in quietly handling and being around your horses, the easier it will be to catch them whenever you want.

The foal will also become accustomed to handling more easily if you regularly put on and take off his halter. In addition, the halter will not become too tight because you will be checking the fit on a daily basis. Foals grow quickly, and if a halter is left on, check it regularly so that it doesn't become so tight that it begins to dig into the skin or rub off the hair.

Just because the young foal is accustomed to wearing his halter doesn't mean that you can attach a rope and lead him around with it. Teaching him to lead will make it much easier to handle your foal, but you still need to be considerate of his vulnerability. You can cause serious damage to the neck or spine if you jerk or pull hard on the foal's head at this early stage.

Make Your Horses Easy to Catch

No doubt you've heard someone say, "He's a great horse, but he's hard to catch." You may even have said it yourself.

Stop and think about it. If the only time you catch your horse is when you want to do something with him, it won't take him long to realize that when you approach him, it means work. Or worse, it may mean something will be done to him, as happens during a visit from the blacksmith or the vet. It doesn't take a particularly smart horse to decide that the way to solve that problem is to avoid being caught.

Consider what your horse is thinking whenever he sees you coming, and make a point of paying short social visits to him *without* catching him. Here are some guidelines.

In the Stall

To establish an unstressful dynamic, always stand quietly at the doorway of the stall and let the horse approach you first. Even though the horse can't get away from you, don't just rush in and grab at him.

Outdoors

Walk out to the pasture or pen so your horse can see you, but don't approach him. Horses are curious creatures and their curiosity will usually get the best of them. If they see you standing by the fence or sitting under a tree reading a magazine, eventually they will come

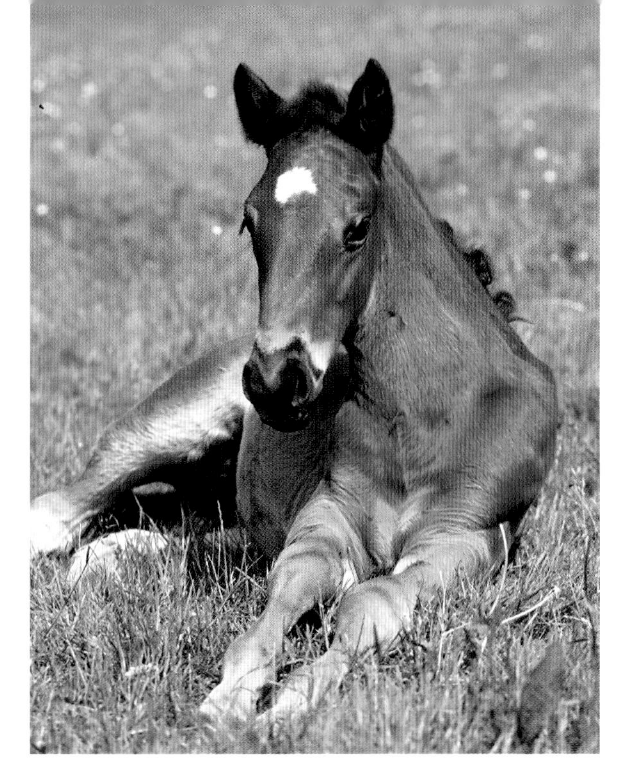

The safest option is not to leave halters on mares and foals when they are turned out.

Why the Left Side?

Although many people handle horses and lead only from the horse's left (or near) side, your horse should learn to accept everything you want to do from his right (or off) side, as well. The tradition of handling horses from the left began long ago, when soldiers wore their swords on their left sides. It was easier to lead and mount the horse from the horse's left so that the sword didn't get in the way. It also made sense because most people are right-handed.

Although handling from the horse's left side has become common practice over the years, there is no legitimate reason now to restrict handling the horse to just one side.

You can, and should, teach your foal to be comfortable with being handled on both sides.

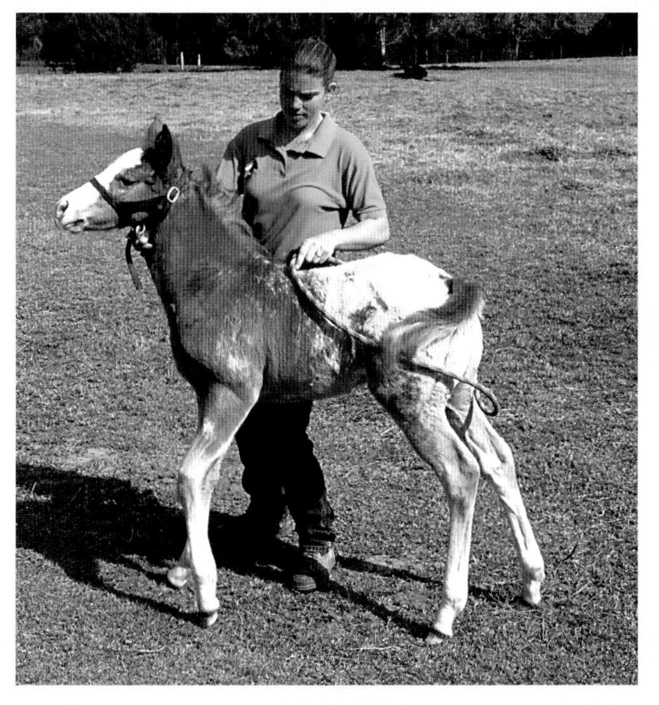

Handle the young foal from both sides so he is comfortable with being handled wherever you are positioned.

over to see what you are doing. Don't try to catch your horse when this happens. Just give him a rub on the neck and offer some kind words. Stay a few minutes and then leave.

Try this "visiting" tactic several times when you don't need to catch the horse for any reason. You can put the halter on if you like and then remove it, or pet the horse and do nothing more.

Then start interspersing these visits with times when you do actually catch the horse. Instead of riding, working, or bringing him in for the blacksmith, give him a good grooming session or hand-walk him and let him graze briefly. Then turn him back into his pen, stall, or paddock.

If you like to give your horse treats, offer them when you are finished with handling him for the day or session. Some people make the mistake of giving a treat every time they go out to catch their horse. A horse will become pushy and aggressive if he expects goodies with your every appearance.

Most horse owners would like to think that their horses consider them friends. With our human friends, we try not to call or visit only when we want something, and we should be as considerate with our equine partners. Call on them just to say hello, and catch them not simply when you want to ride or because the vet is coming.

If you have a new foal, it's natural to want to spend plenty of time with him, especially when he's an adorable baby. Just be sure to set the right tone for your relationship from the very beginning. Catch and handle him frequently, but don't halter him every time you initiate contact. Let some visits be purely social. Allow him to approach you whenever possible, and always insist that he respect your space, no matter how friendly and people oriented he is.

"Mouthing" Behavior

You may notice the young foal making a funny movement with his mouth if he is scared or startled or when a horse other than his mother approaches him. This rapid "chomping" motion is a submissive action similar to a puppy rolling over on his back and exposing his belly to another dog. This is the foal's way of saying, "I'm submissive to you. Don't hurt me!"

Foals have distinctly different personalities and this will play a role in how the foal relates to you. Some foals are quite bold at a young age and will walk right up to you, even when this means walking away from "mom." Other foals are shy and will hang back, trying to hide behind their dam. Once you have a feel for your foal's mood and personality, you will begin to learn how to best interact with him.

Safe Methods of Restraint

It's a good idea to know how to restrain the foal safely should he need to be held — for a veterinary procedure, perhaps, or for your examination or handling.

First, cradle him around his chest with one arm and, with your other hand, grasp the base of his tail, holding it upright . Holding the tail this way will help restrain the foal. Don't be too forceful, or he will struggle or sink to the ground. Another way to restrain him is to stand the foal against the stall wall, using your body to keep him close against the wall. If your head is above the foal's head, he can jerk it up and pop you under the chin. *Always be sure your head is positioned above his back, not over his head.*

Early Lessons before Leading

Among a group of horses, the dominant, or **alpha,** animal uses physical actions and body language to make the others move according to his or her will. The horse that moves the most is usually the lowest in the pecking order. The alpha horse often has to do no more than flatten his ears and appear threatening to make the more submissive horses move. As you control your foal's movements when handling him, he begins to consider you the leader of his herd, and this is where the all-important element of respect comes into play.

Lay the foundation for leading with the following simple lessons taught in the stall. The foal can be haltered, but you will not be controlling him with the halter at this point. Have someone else hold the mare so you can concentrate on handling the foal.

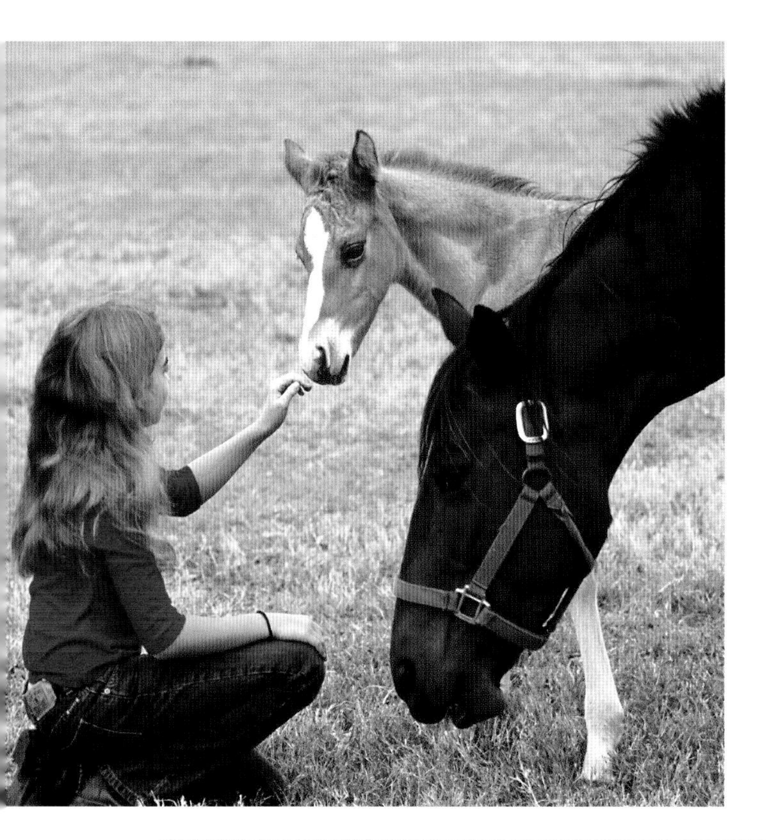

Moving Away from Pressure

Standing beside the foal on either his left side or his right, press your fingertips against the base of his neck, just above the chest. Keep pressing until he backs up or leans back. Immediately release pressure when the foal responds this way. It will not take long for him to learn to move away from pressure, a lesson that will be valuable for the rest of his life. Do this several times, until the foal learns to back up at the slightest pressure of your fingertips.

Still standing beside the foal, put your hand on his hindquarters, just below his tail. Use steady pressure until the foal moves forward. You want the foal to step forward when he feels light pressure from behind. This is the first step in teaching the foal to lead. Soon you will be using a butt rope, instead of your hand, to provide this incentive to move forward.

Moving Sideways from Pressure

Once the foal is easily moving forward and backward from hand pressure, it's time to teach him to move sideways, or laterally.

Stand next to the foal on his left side with your left arm under his neck to keep him from moving forward. Reach over his back with your right arm and press your fingertips into his **flank,** the lower part of his side just in front of his hind leg. Keep pressing with your fingers until he moves his body toward you. Be sure you don't block his movement. You are conditioning the foal to move sideways away from pressure. His front feet should stay in the same place, but his hindquarters will move sideways, away from the pressure of your hand. Switch your position and do this on both sides.

After a few short lessons, your foal should be moving forward, backward, and sideways from your hand pressure. At this point, you're ready to teach him to lead.

The foal can bond with humans as well as his dam.

Lessons in Leading

You may be tempted to let the foal follow loose behind his mother when you lead the pair in and out of the stall. This might work fine in the first days, when the newborn is determined to stick close to his mother's side. It can spell trouble, however, when you have an independent foal who decides to run off and go adventuring, leaving you holding on to an upset, prancing mare.

Avoid potential accidents by handling the foal from day one and by always leading him in and out of the stall. This will mean you need two people, one for the mare and one for the foal, but it's safer than trying to lead both mare and foal by yourself or leaving the foal to run loose.

Leading with a Halter

Start teaching the foal to lead within the safe confines of the stall. And be sure to have a second person there to handle the mare.

Put the halter on the foal and, standing on his left side, use your left hand on the halter's cheekpiece to guide him. Urge him forward by exerting gentle pressure on his hindquarters, as you taught him previously. Using this method, move him in a circle around the stall. Switch sides and handle him in the same way from his right side.

You can begin leading the foal in and out of the stall in this manner once he is responding well inside the enclosed area. Always have someone else lead the mare so you do not have to try to hold both horses. Attempting to manage both mare and foal by yourself is asking for trouble, especially if the foal tries to run backward or leap forward. When someone else is handling the mare, you can use the cradling method to hold the foal if he gets rambunctious.

Leading with a Lead Rope

Again, use the confines of the stall to introduce the foal to leading with a lead rope. Your lesson will be the same as leading by the halter cheekpiece, except you hold the lead rope just below the snap where it attaches to the halter. Use your other hand to provide light pressure on the foal's hindquarters to encourage him to move forward while you *gently* pull forward on the lead rope. (Remember, you can damage the foal's neck and/or spine if you are forceful.) If you have taught the foal to move away from the pressure of your hand, it should be easy to guide him around the stall, and he will quickly adapt to following the direction of your hand on the lead rope.

Once your foal has advanced to this step, change to a butt rope to continue teaching him to lead.

You can make a butt rope to teach the new foal to lead.

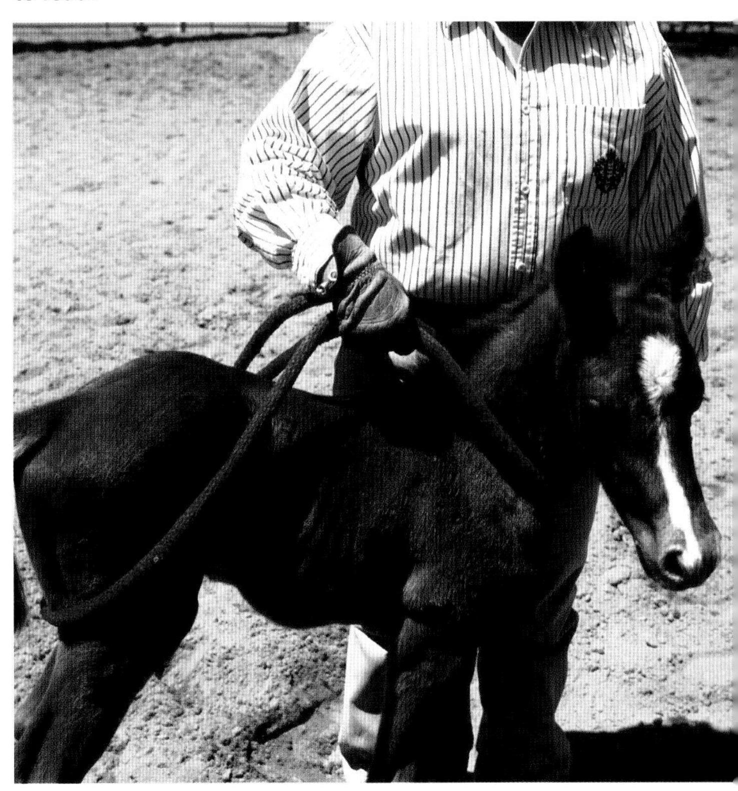

Leading with a Butt Rope

A butt rope can be useful in teaching the foal not only to lead but also to stand quietly for veterinary and blacksmith procedures. Many people use the end of the lead rope as a makeshift butt rope to encourage the foal to lead, or you can make your own butt rope from a separate rope. (See box.) As usual, you will need an assistant during this lesson.

To use the butt rope, stand close to the foal and cradle him so he can't move away. Have your assistant slip one loop of the butt rope over the foal's head and neck. Then figure-eight the loop over the middle of the foal's back and slip the back loop down over his hindquarters under his tail. When you put the butt rope on the foal, the metal clamp should be near where the rope figure-eights over his back.

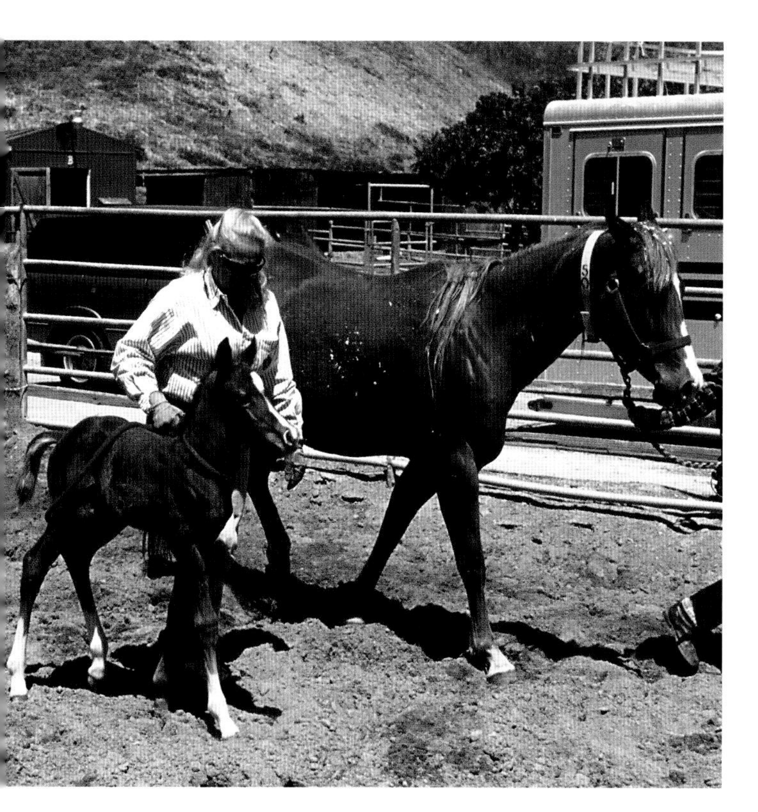

Using the butt rope will help the new foal learn to lead without putting too much pressure or pull on his head and neck.

The rope shouldn't be tight, nor should it be overly loose and dangle below the hocks. It should rest just below the foal's hindquarters. Hold on to the rope at the figure eight over the foal's back, just behind the **withers,** where the neck and mane end. This will keep you close to the foal, giving you good leverage and control.

Lead him from his left side with your left hand on his halter and your right hand holding the butt rope. He will adapt easily to leading with only a lead rope once he catches on.

When you are ready to turn the foal loose, slip the butt rope off his hindquarters. Then slip off the end that is around his shoulders and head. Finally, turn him loose altogether by removing or letting go of the halter.

After the foal is leading well with the butt rope, gradually exert less pressure against his hindquarters. The amount of time this will take depends on the individual foal and on how frequently you handle him. You can continue using the butt rope as a "security blanket" until he is leading well with only a lead rope. Remember, you can also slip the end of a regular lead rope around the foal's hindquarters to act as a butt rope whenever he needs reinforcement.

Turn Out

During the first few days after foaling, it is especially helpful to the mare to spend time outside and moving around. This encourages her uterus to flush out. It is normal for the mare to have some discharge from the vulva during the first week as part of her body's natural cleanup process after giving birth.

For the first few days to two weeks of your foal's life, turn him out with his mother in a safe enclosure separate from other horses. After this period, unless the foal has problems or your vet instructs otherwise, it is usually safe to turn the two of them out with other mares and young foals. Socially, it's important for the foal

Making Your Own Butt Rope

Use soft cotton or poly rope, such as lead ropes are made of. The rope should be no less than half an inch thick but no more than one inch thick.

1. To determine how long the rope should be, hold it from the foal's nose to tail without stretching it tight. Allow it to drape slightly. Double this amount and cut the rope. For the average foal, you will need about six feet of rope.
2. Tape or burn both ends of the rope to prevent unraveling.
3. Make a loop by bringing both ends together and closing them tight with a metal rope clamp.

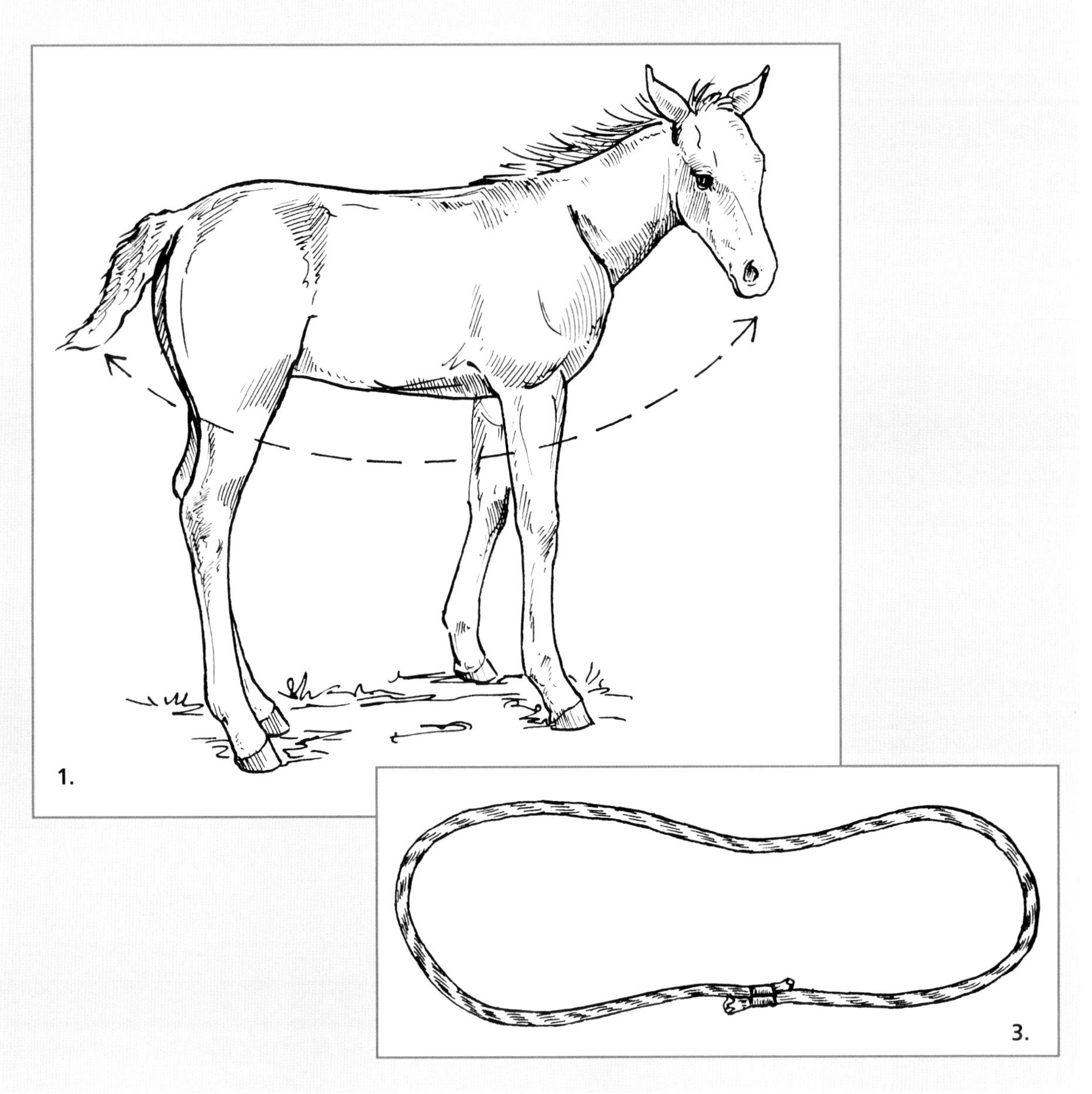

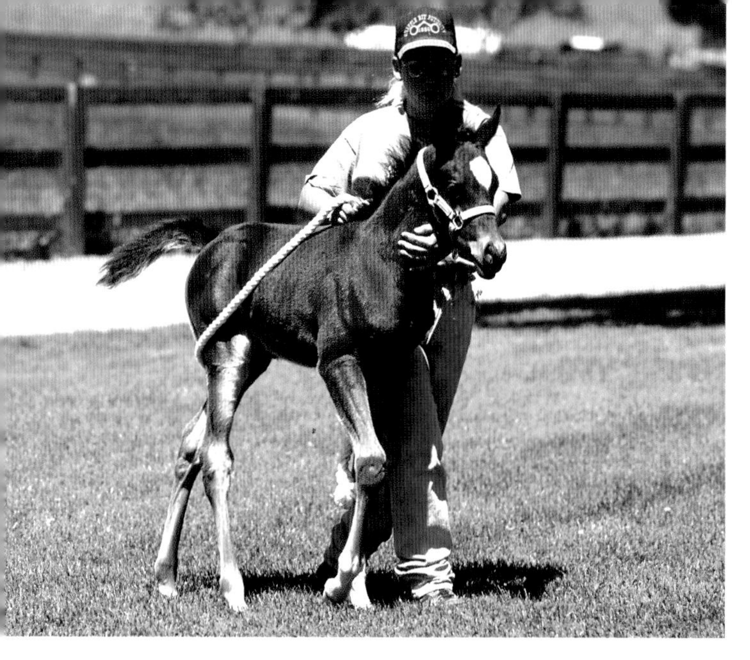

You can use the end of the lead rope to encourage the foal to move forward.

to have playmates roughly his same age. If there aren't other mares and foals, do not turn out mother and son with geldings or other mares without babies, as these horses may act dangerously aggressive toward the foal.

The safest method of turning out with other horses is to pair your mare and foal with one other mare and foal at first. The other mare should not be overly dominant or bossy; ideally, she will be a mare that your mare is already familiar with. If there are other mares and foals on the farm, it's usually best to increase the herd size gradually by adding mares and foals over the course of a few days rather than turning out everyone at once.

When introducing a new mare and foal to the group, don't release them until the others have settled down and moved off to graze. If the rest of the herd is milling around the gate or crowding in, don't turn loose the new mare and foal. The other horses will invariably approach the mare and foal to make their introductions, but the newcomers should be provided with enough space to get away from the herd's curiosity if they choose.

When you introduce a mare and foal into a group, it is helpful to put out an extra pile of hay at feeding time. The horses will naturally jostle each other and change eating spots, and this way there is always a spot for the "displaced" mare and foal to go.

Whether you are turning out the mare and foal by themselves or with a group, remember the safety tip of turning the mare to face her foal before you let her loose (see page 48). After the first few times outside, turn the mare to face the baby, then release the foal first.

Keep a close eye on the two — the foal can become exhausted quickly if the mare runs around or won't settle down and keeps walking. For the first week, try to turn out twice during the day, rather than for one long stretch.

Because the new foal is physically vulnerable, don't force him to endure temperature extremes or wet weather. Always make sure there is adequate shade if the weather is warm, and bring the mare and foal inside if the weather turns chilly, damp, or rainy. He will soon become hardier with age, but a new foal, particularly in the first two weeks of life, is a fragile creature.

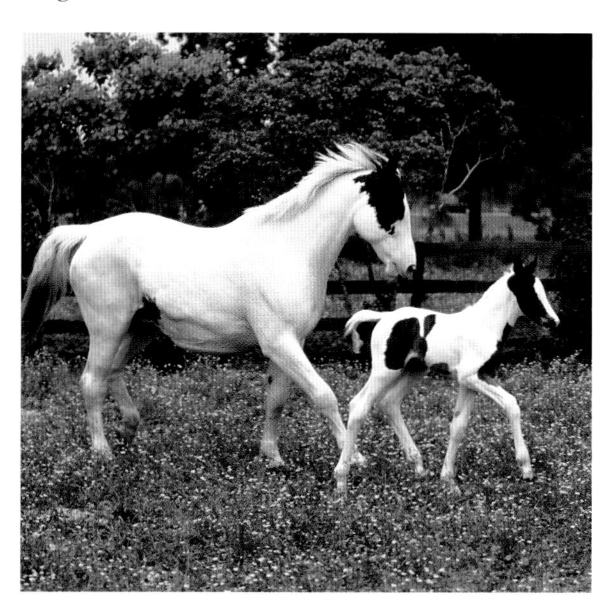

Time outside in their own paddock is beneficial to the new foal and his dam.

Things to Watch For in the First Weeks

Several common situations will arise during the first weeks of your foal's life. It's advisable to learn about them before they happen.

Foal Heat

Foal heat refers not to any temperature issues with the foal, but rather to the first heat cycle the mare goes through, which takes place 6 to 12 days after foaling and lasts for about 4 days.

Typically, the foal will develop scours (diarrhea) during the mare's foal heat. The old theory was that the mare's heat cycle caused changes in her milk that resulted in the foal developing scours. Veterinarians now believe that foal-heat diarrhea is part of the foal's natural development of normal intestinal flora and adjustment to eating solid food.

The typical foal with foal-heat scours does not exhibit a fever and will continue to nurse normally. He will appear healthy with the exception of having loose, runny stools.

Keep a close eye on him during this time, because the danger of scours is dehydration. The foal's hindquarters will become irritated, or "scalded," and can lose hair due to the diarrhea. Wash and dry the area, then coat it two or three times daily with a layer of petroleum jelly, Preparation H, or a zinc oxide/ lanolin product such as Desitin to soothe the skin. This will also help prevent hair loss.

Several supplement products contain egg protein, thought to prevent or decrease diarrhea. Ask your vet for her recommendation. She may suggest treating foal-heat scours with Pepto Bismol or Kaopectate, either of which slows the diarrhea and helps the foal feel better. She will prescribe the dosage and frequency. To administer liquid medication, put some in a clean syringe, without a needle, and squirt a small amount at a time into the foal's mouth.

Some veterinarians recommend that treatment for foal-heat scours routinely include a simple dewormer, such as a fenbendazole product (brand names include Safeguard and Panacur), given at an appropriate dose, in case the foal has ingested parasite eggs/larvae. This

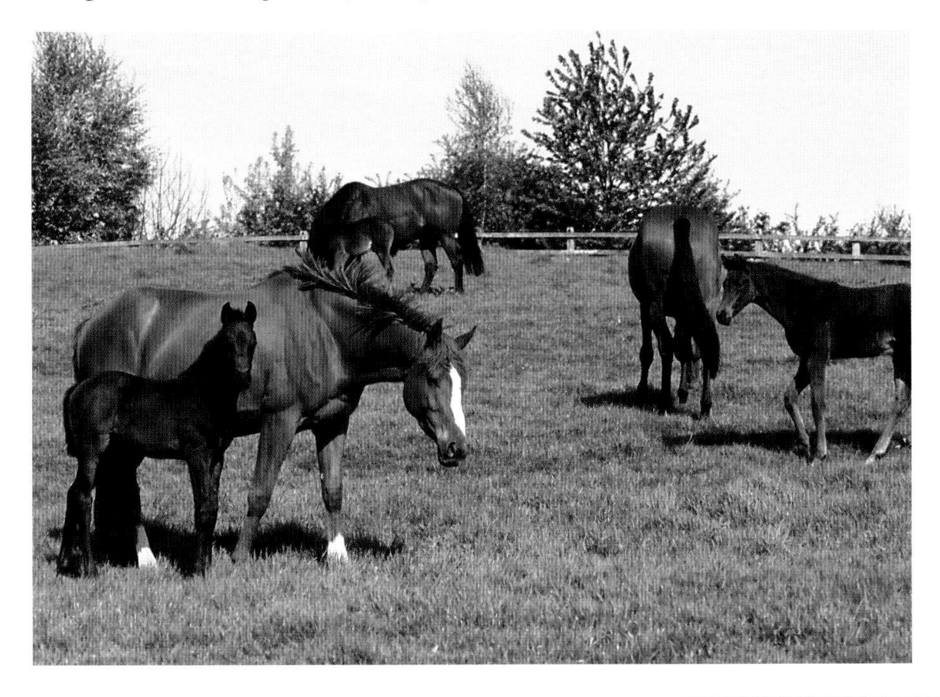

In a group, young foals will often stay close to their dams. As they get older and braver, they will venture off to play with each other.

is especially appropriate if there has been a parasite problem with other horses on the farm.

If the foal has scours and runs a fever or acts dull and loses interest in nursing, he needs prompt veterinary attention. The diarrhea may be a symptom of something other than the mare's foal heat.

Eating Manure

New foals will often eat manure. This behavior, known as **coprophagia,** may be unsavory to humans, but it is normal for the young foal. One theory is that this introduces bacteria naturally found in the environment into the foal's gastrointestinal tract.

Veterinary Exam for Mare

Your mare should have a reproductive exam seven to nine days after foaling, whether or not you are breeding her back this season. Some vets use a **speculum,** a device that allows them to see inside the mare's reproductive tract, to make sure the birth canal and cervix look normal after the recent delivery.

After examining the mare, your vet will tell you whether she requires any treatment. If you plan to breed your mare back this season, the veterinarian will work with you to determine when the mare is in heat and most likely to conceive.

Nursing and Eating Solid Food

Take a close look at the mouth of the newborn foal and you will see just pink gums. The foal's first teeth, the central incisors, will erupt within the first few days or week of life. The middle incisors come through in four to six weeks, and the corner incisors will erupt in four to six months. An easy way to remember this is 6-6-6: 6 days for central incisors, 6 weeks for middle incisors, and 6 months for corner incisors.

Foals grow quickly and should gain between one and three pounds a day. By the time your foal is a few weeks old, he will nurse only about once an hour, and the time between nursing periods will increase as he gets older.

When they are just a few days old, many foals will show interest in and try to eat their mother's hay and grain. Don't try to restrict a foal from eating with his mother. It is normal for him to start grazing and nibbling grass now. Although he may be eating some of his mother's feed, his main source of nutrition is still the mare's milk. By the time the foal is several weeks old, offer him his own feed (see chapter 7).

During the first two months of lactation, the mare will consume about 3 percent of her body weight in feed and produce about 3 percent of her weight in milk each day. An average-sized mare produces 3 to 4 gallons of milk daily. Peak milk production and quality occurs about a month after foaling and slowly declines from there. Milk alone will meet the foal's nutrient requirements during that first month after birth.

About two months after foaling, both milk production and the protein and energy content of the mare's milk decrease markedly. By this time the foal is already eating grass, hay, and grain, so he is obtaining nutrition from these sources and not just from his mother's milk.

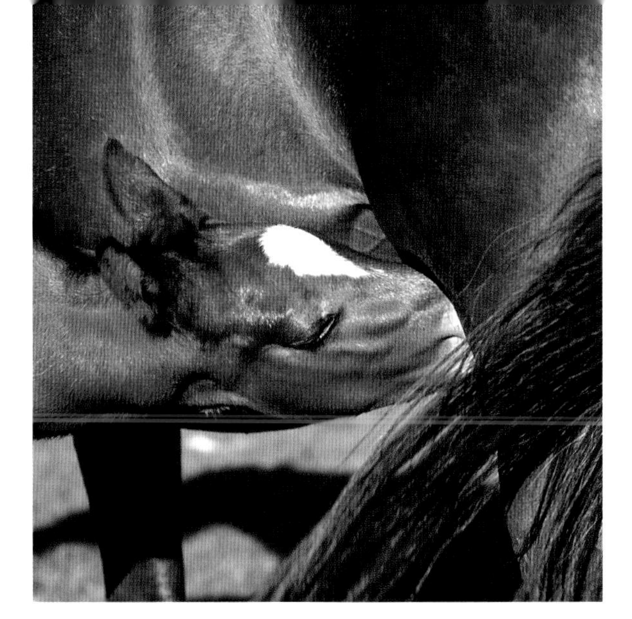

For the first weeks of life, his mother's milk is the foal's main source of nutrition.

Feeding the Lactating Mare

Proper nutrition for the broodmare plays a critical role for both mother and foal and cannot be overestimated. Nutritional demands on her are greatest for the first three months of lactation.

Immediately after foaling, the mare's energy requirements increase by as much as 90 percent, and her protein requirements increase by 50 percent. If she does not receive the proper diet during this time, she will lose weight and body condition in order to produce milk for her foal. This can also make it more difficult for her to become pregnant if she is bred again.

To produce plenty of quality milk, the mare needs unlimited access to water and a balanced ration of adequate roughage, protein, vitamins, and minerals. Rough-stemmed **forage** (grass and/or hay) should always make up the bulk of her diet. **Concentrates** (commercial feed ration/grain) provide nutrients in a dense form, but the horse needs forage for her digestive system to function properly. The only reason to add a concentrate to the daily diet is to make up the difference between the nutrients in the forage and the requirements of the individual horse. Once you decide on the forage/hay source, balance it by choosing the correct concentrate.

Early Lactation (First 3 Months)

Forage: 1–2% of mare's body weight
Concentrate: 1–2% of mare's body weight
Total daily intake should be approximately 2–3% of mare's body weight

Important! The mare's forage intake should never be less than 1% of her body weight, even if you are increasing the concentrate. She could colic or founder without enough forage.

Example (adjust to your specific mare's weight and needs):

- 1,000-pound mare × 1 to 2% of body weight in forage = 10 to 20 pounds forage (1 to 2 pounds forage per 100 pounds body weight)
- 1,000-pound mare × 1 to 2% body weight in concentrate = 10 to 20 pounds concentrate (1 to 2 pounds concentrate per 100 pounds body weight)

Total feed ration: approximately 20–30 pounds/day

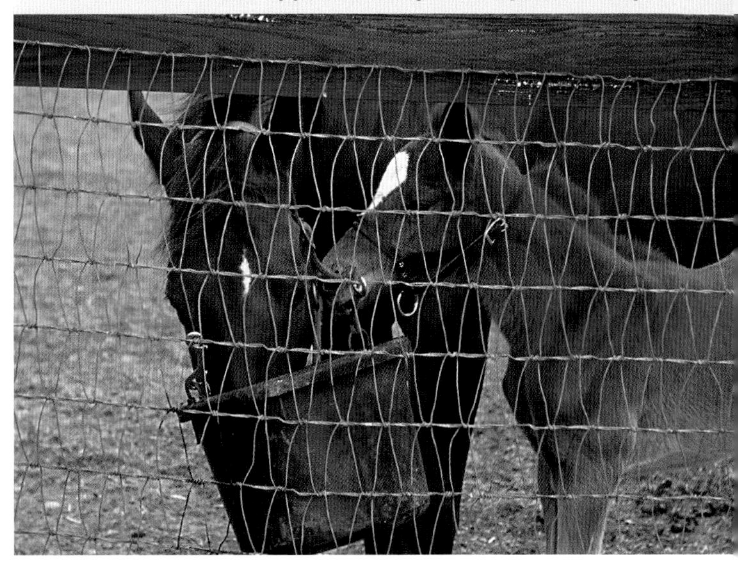

It's normal for the young foal to show some interest in his mother's feed even when he is just a few days old.

For example, if you are feeding the lactating mare good-quality, high-protein legume hay, such as alfalfa, or a legume/grass mix hay that is high in alfalfa, such as alfalfa/timothy mix, a commercial 12 percent protein concentrate designed for lactating mares should be adequate. If the mare is on grass pasture or is being fed grass hay, such as orchard, timothy, or coastal, a higher percentage of protein (14 to 16 percent, or even 18 percent) is needed in the concentrate.

Look for a nutritionally balanced commercial feed designed for pregnant/lactating mares. It is tempting to add supplements to your mare's diet, but do this only on your veterinarian's specific recommendation. Commercial feed is already balanced. Follow the feeding recommendations on the bag, and consult your veterinarian if you have any questions.

Some mares are easy keepers and don't require as much feed as others, so there is no one-size-fits-all chart when it comes to feeding. For example, Thoroughbreds typically require more feed than Quarter Horses. Feeding charts offer a general starting point when deciding how much to feed, but even among the same breed, horses' needs can vary dramatically, so adjust the amount of feed for each individual horse.

The horse's digestive system is designed for almost constant eating, so always divide feed into two, preferably more, feedings per day.

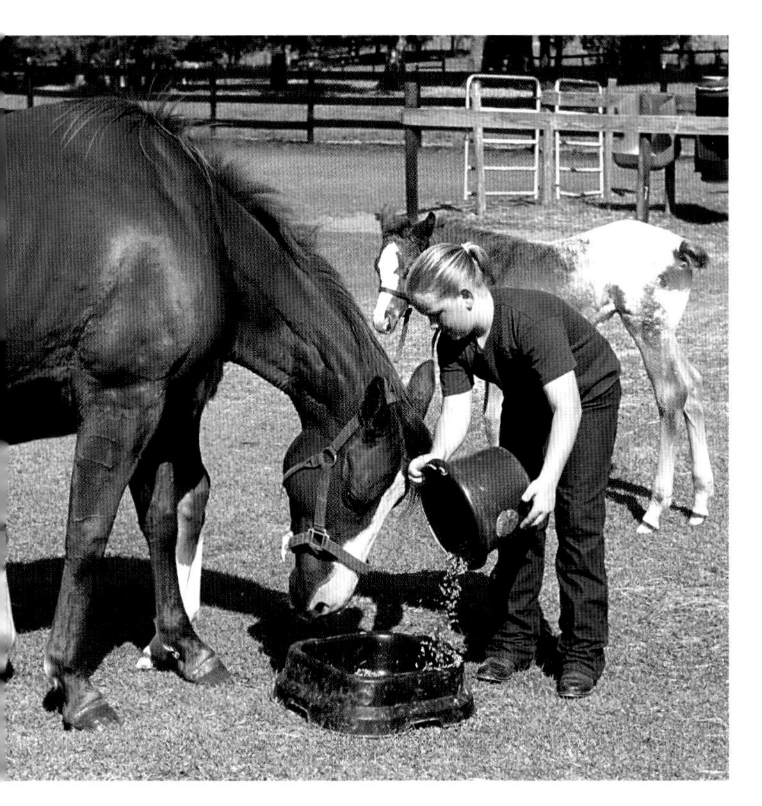

The nursing mare must receive adequate feed in order to produce milk without losing weight and body condition.

To-Do List

First Weeks

- ☐ First day: put halter on new foal and then remove.
- ☐ Check the mare's udder twice a day to be sure foal is nursing normally.
- ☐ Mare's foal heat (anywhere from 6 to 12 days after foaling). Keep an eye on diarrhea of foal; treat if necessary.
- ☐ Time outside for mare and foal (alone) for first week or two, then turn out with other mares and foals unless vet says otherwise. Avoid turning out during temperature extremes and wet weather for first several weeks.
- ☐ Postfoaling reproductive veterinary exam for mare around 7 or 9 days.
- ☐ Handle foal daily.
- ☐ Teach foal to lead.

7

One to Three Months

Learning and Growing

Prepare to witness a variety of changes as your foal grows and blossoms during his first three months. By now, he may be gaining as much as 3 pounds per day. As prey animals, horses have to mature fast physically for survival. The average healthy young horse gains 90 percent or more of his full adult size in just the first 24 months of life.

Nutrition for the First Months

Although the foal will nibble at his dam's feed during the first weeks of life, all the nutrition he needs is contained in his mother's milk. Starting at about one month of age, however, the foal needs more nutrition than his mother's milk alone can provide. At this stage, it is important that the foal have access to feed designed to meet his individual needs. For example, the levels of copper and zinc in a mare's milk are low. By two months, the foal should be eating his own ration, in addition to his mother's milk, in order to maintain optimal growth.

The horse's first year is a crucial period of development. Proper nutrition is critical now, because the young animal is building a lifetime foundation of bone and muscle. The majority of bone growth occurs between the ages of three months before birth to about nine months of age. Maximum muscle growth takes place from about 2 months to 22 months.

Weak bones and joints will affect the horse's soundness and athletic ability as an adult. If a young horse doesn't receive adequate nutrition and exercise during his first year, it will be impossible to correct deficiencies in bone or joint development when he is older.

His mother's feed is not formulated for the growing foal's needs. Commercial feeds for foals are more concentrated because young horses can't eat the same volume as adult horses. Look for a high-quality feed (typically 14 to 16 percent protein) formulated specifically for growing foals with the proper balance of vitamins and minerals. Calcium, phosphorus, copper, and zinc are especially important for the foal at this stage of growth.

Offer the foal his own feed at about 1 month of age, but don't expect him to eat much yet. A pound a day is the *maximum* the young foal should eat. This amount is approximately ½ to 1 percent of his body weight. *Don't feed foals more than one pound of feed per month of age.* The foal's stomach is relatively small, so divide feed into two — or preferably three — feedings per day.

If you are feeding the mare and foal in the stall, provide the foal with a separate feeder. Foal feeders that feature a small opening to keep the mare from stealing her baby's ration are available.

Some farms with multiple foals have a **creep feeder** in the field. This is a pen built to keep out mares while allowing foals to walk under a top rail, or through a narrow opening, to reach the manger or the feed trough inside. Hay can be offered to foals in a creep feeder, but it is not recommended to feed a grain ration this way. Invariably, the bigger, bossier foals eat more and it is impossible to keep track of how much each individual foal is actually consuming. The most reliable method of feeding foals is to provide them with their own feeder in the stall or pen.

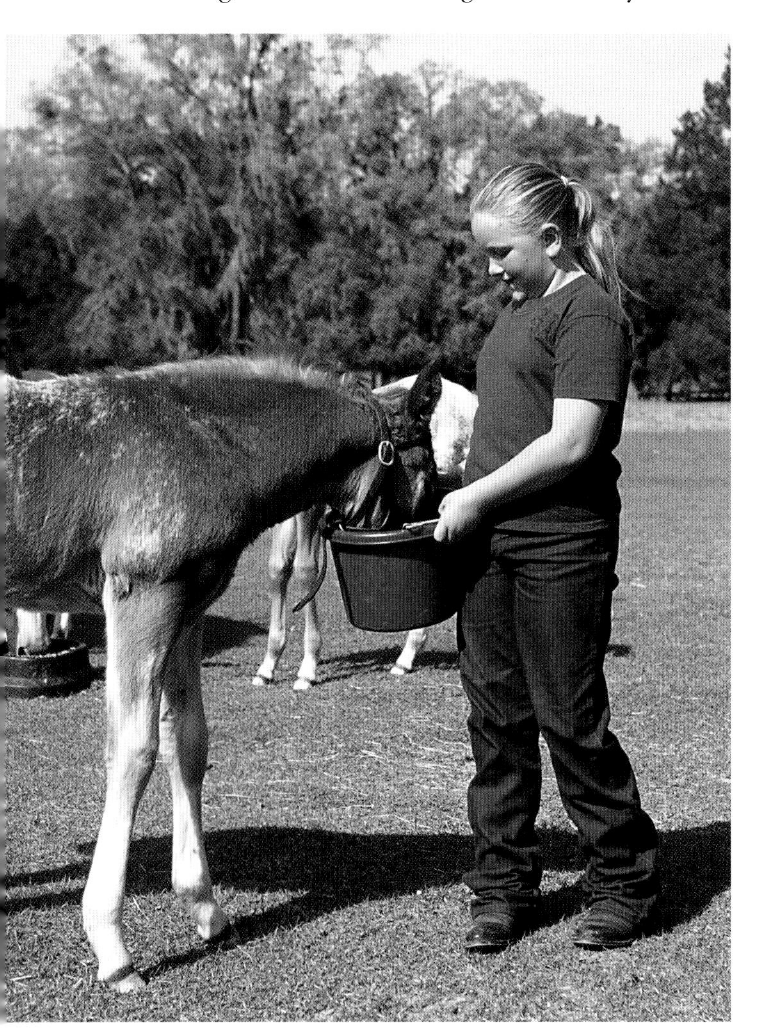

Feed a quality ration designed specifically for his needs.

Don't offer grain to the foal **free choice** (as much as the horse wants to eat). Feed can spoil or be contaminated by birds or other disease-carrying wild creatures. Put out only enough grain for each feeding and remove any uneaten feed between meals. It is important to remember that unlike humans, dogs, cats, and most other animals, horses cannot vomit. If the foal eats too much or eats spoiled feed, it cannot relieve discomfort by "getting sick."

Make available to the foal plenty of high-quality pasture or hay. Unless you are feeding straight alfalfa, you can offer hay free choice so the foal can eat as much and whenever he wants. The best hay for growing foals is a mixture of alfalfa and grass hay, such as orchard or timothy.

Protein Isn't the Problem!

In the past, too much protein in the young horse's feed was blamed for developmental orthopedic disease (DOD). Studies later proved this untrue. A number of factors can be responsible for DOD, including genetics, exercise, nutrition, and rapid growth rate. Feeding a

Mare Nutrition

The mare's nutritional needs are greatest during these early months of lactation. Refer to the feeding information in chapter 6 to make sure she is receiving adequate nutrition to produce enough quality milk for her rapidly growing foal.

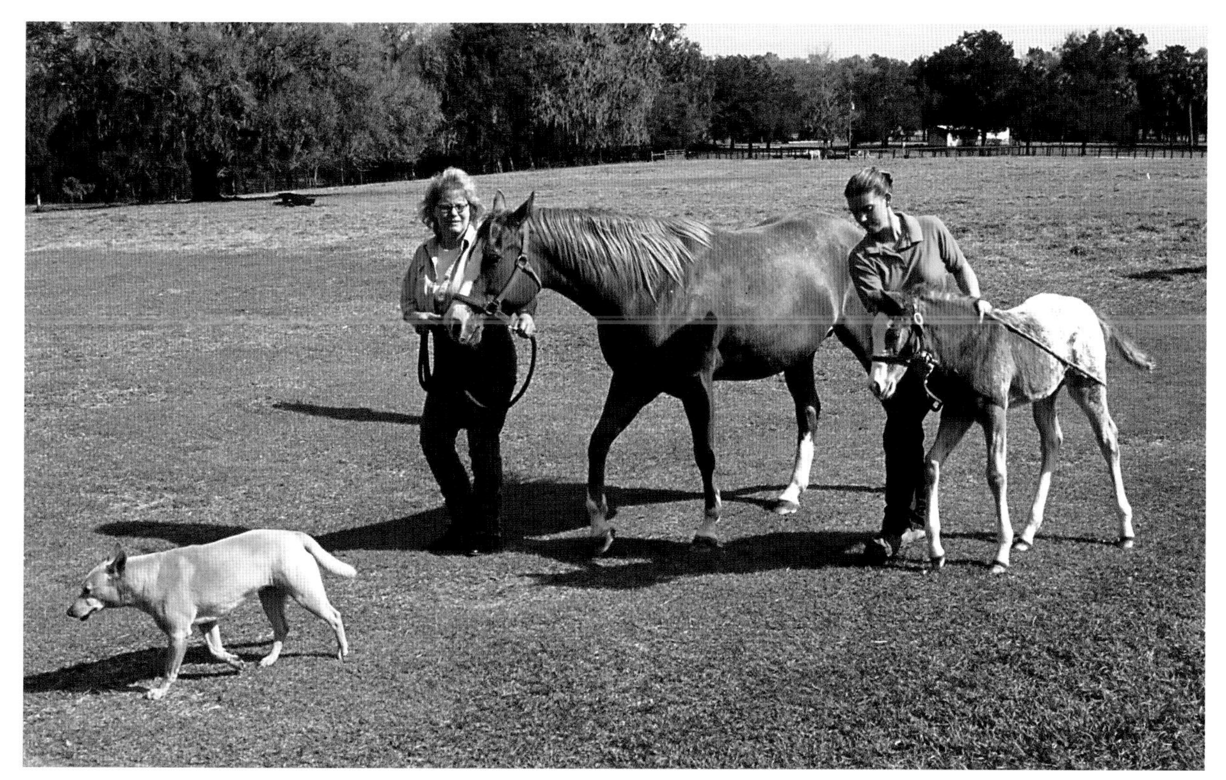

Use a butt rope to encourage the foal to move forward.

high-calorie ration and unbalanced amounts of vitamins and minerals can also cause DOD.

Much more than just an energy source, protein is actually necessary to sustain life. If all the water and fat were removed from the horse's body, the remainder would be about 80 percent pure protein. And every 45 days the protein content of the muscle cells in a horse's body is replaced by new protein. Most of the protein in the horse's diet comes from forage, which is why wild horses can survive without any grain.

Handling and Leading

Your foal's unique personality will be more and more evident as he grows. By handling him regularly, you will build on the trust and respect you have already established.

If you're haltering and leading the foal on a regular basis during his first three months, it won't take long before you'll be able to lead him without using a butt rope or lead rope behind his hindquarters. There is nothing wrong with using the butt rope or lead rope for encouragement, however, if you feel you need it (see page 64).

It is tempting to allow the foal to follow along as you lead his mother, but don't slip into this habit. As the foal gets older and more independent, he will want to run off from his mother to go exploring, which is fine if he's in the pasture but not when you're holding on to the mare and the foal is galloping around the barn on his own. A loose foal can get into trouble or hurt himself in a matter of seconds.

The safest plan is always to have two people available whenever you need to move the mare and foal. It can be dangerous to try leading both mare and foal by yourself.

The more you practice leading the foal, the better he will behave. Always hold the foal's lead rope within a few inches of the halter. Don't give him a lot of extra rope when you are leading; instead, coil the excess in your left hand so it doesn't drag on the ground. *Never* wrap a lead rope around your hand, wrist, arm, or body in any way. People have been dragged to death after making this mistake.

It is best not to leave a halter on your foal. If, however, for some reason you decide to leave on a halter, use *only* a leather halter, which should break loose if the foal catches it on something. Check the fit of the halter at least once a week to be sure it isn't too snug and isn't rubbing the hair on the foal's face.

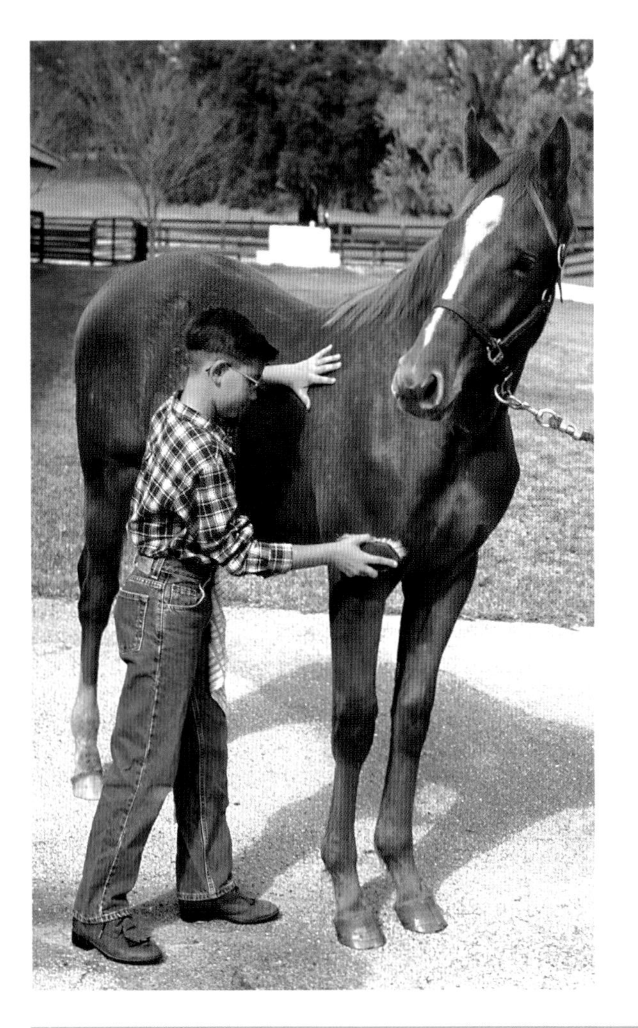

Whenever you are working around a horse, stay close to him. It helps if you keep one hand on the horse at all times, so he is aware of where you are.

Get Grooming!

Grooming sessions are an enjoyable way to spend time with your foal and reinforce the idea that you are allowed to touch him all over his body. They also provide an excellent opportunity to teach him simple lessons that will come in handy when he is older, such as backing up and moving sideways and forward.

You can groom the foal in the stall after he has eaten. Some horses don't mind if you do this while they are eating, but others will act defensively. Give the foal his private time to eat so you can have his focused attention while you groom him.

If the mare is likely to move around the stall, you may want to tie her so she stands still. Give the mare a grooming session with the foal loose in the stall. Once you are finished with the mare, put a lead rope on the foal, even though you are not going to tie him at this point.

Start the lesson by slowly and gently rubbing the end of the lead rope over the foal's body, belly, neck, and face. The more relaxed he is about equipment at a young age, the easier it will be to introduce him to tack later.

Use a rubber currycomb to rub in small circles on the body. This will raise dirt off the skin and stimulate circulation; most horses love the sensation. Don't use a currycomb on legs or sensitive areas. The face, legs, flanks, and belly are the most tender places. Don't use a stiff brush on the foal at all. Use a soft-bristled brush on sensitive areas, as the idea is always to make grooming a pleasant experience.

Follow the currying with a soft-bristled brush to knock off the dirt and smooth the coat. Always brush the hair in the direction it grows. Use a soft brush on his face, and don't forget the inside of the ears. Clean the nose with a paper towel, which is more sanitary than a grooming rag. A human hairbrush is easier on manes and tails than is a comb, as it tends to pull out less hair.

To finish, run a "rub rag," or terry cloth hand towel, over the entire body to remove any dust and to add shine.

In every grooming session, run your hands up and down each leg and over the foal's body to learn what every part normally feels like. Once you get accustomed to this practice, it will be easy to notice if there are any swollen or warm areas, small cuts, abrasions, or bumps on the skin.

Finally, pick up and clean out your foal's feet regularly. This will make hoof trimming much easier on both him and the blacksmith.

Gently squeeze the back of the leg above the ankle until the foal picks up that foot. He will quickly learn to give you his hoof as soon as you barely touch his leg. When you are done, set the foot down; don't just drop it abruptly, as this can throw the foal off balance.

During the grooming session, take advantage of opportunities to make the foal back up a few steps. As you did in those first lessons (see chapter 6), press your fingertips against the base of his neck just above the chest. As soon as he backs away, release this pressure. If you want the foal to associate voice commands with what you are asking him to do, repeat the command *Back* in an even voice and praise him when he responds.

Ask the foal to move sideways in both directions by pressing your fingertips into his flank. To use a voice command, say *Move over* when you press your fingertips into his right flank to make him move left. To make him move right, press your fingertips into his left flank.

The command *Whoa* means you want the foal to stand still.

The foal will soon learn what you are asking of him; these lessons will stay with him for a lifetime, making it easier and safer to handle him on the ground later.

Grooming Tools

You can use many of the same grooming tools on the foal that you use on the mare, but don't use a stiff brush on a foal. Keep your brushes and equipment clean by regularly washing with soap and water, then air drying. Periodically disinfect them after washing, using the same product you use to disinfect the stall. Allow equipment to dry thoroughly before using anything on the horse.
Your grooming box should contain:

- Soft-bristled body brush
- Medium-bristled body brush
- Rubber currycomb
- Comb or human hairbrush for manes and tails
- Rub rag or terry cloth hand towel
- Hoof pick
- Sturdy paper towels
- Coat conditioner/mane detangler, such as Show Sheen
- Shampoo
- Sweat scraper

Time Outside

Young foals should never have forced vigorous exercise, but they can be outside as much as possible unless a medical condition requires confinement.

It is generally recommended that foals be turned out in a pasture where they can graze, play, and rest for the majority of the day. Foals that are kept inside or in situations where exercise is restricted can end up with poor bone growth and development. Allow foals and their mothers as much time outdoors as possible, except in extreme weather conditions.

If your mare and foal are pastured with other mares and foals, this is an ideal opportunity for the foal to socialize with his peers. It's entertaining to watch the foals interact, play together, and learn to mutually groom each other.

Mutual grooming is one example of healthy social interaction.

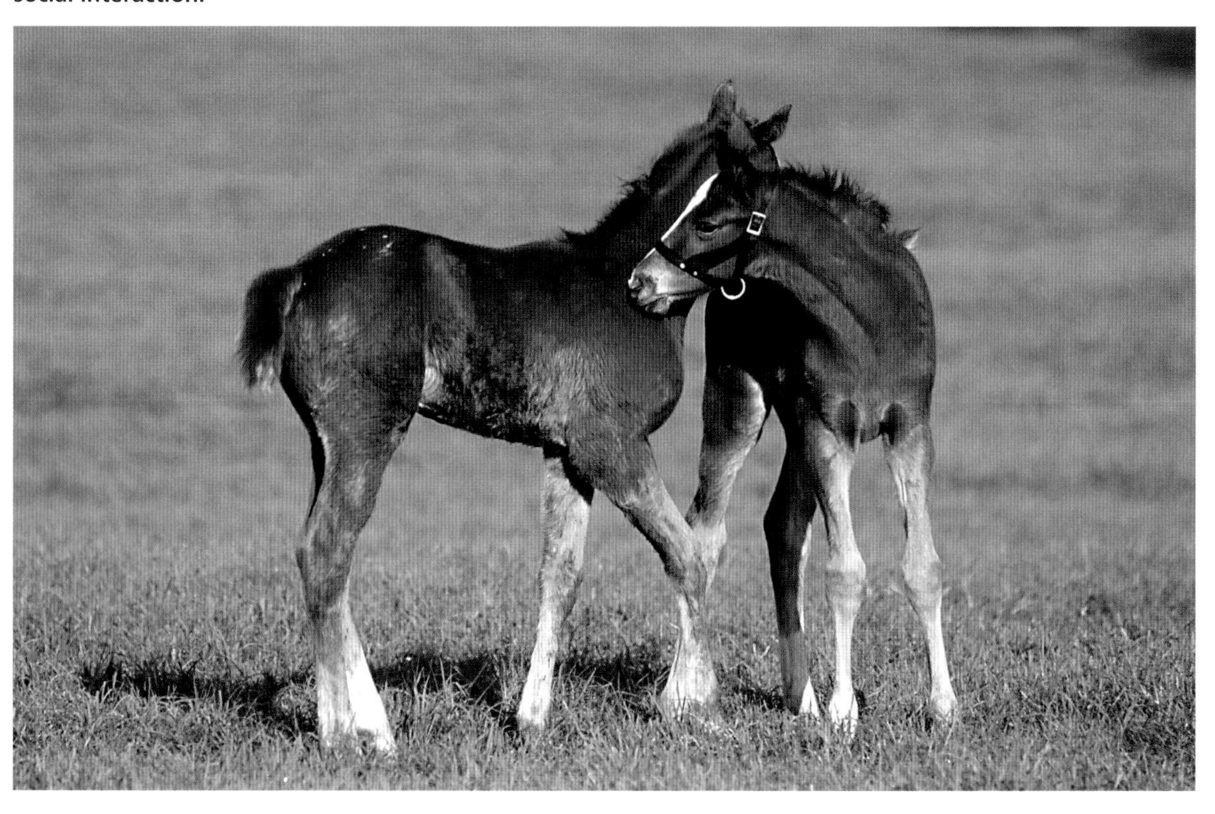

Health Issues in the First Three Months

Make sure your foal has the most advantageous start in life by keeping him in good health. Always consult your veterinarian if you have any concerns about specific health issues in a growing foal.

First Vaccinations

If your mare was properly vaccinated during pregnancy, her foal will be protected from these diseases during his first few months of life. **Passive immunity** is the protection the foal receives by drinking the mare's colostrum within the first hours of life. The mare can pass on these protective maternal antibodies only if she has been properly vaccinated and receives booster vaccinations four to six weeks before foaling.

If the foal is vaccinated while the maternal antibodies are still active in his system, the vaccine will not be effective. The length of time the antibodies remain in the foal's body as protection can vary, so it is important to discuss with the veterinarian when to start the foal's vaccination program.

Many vets recommend giving the first vaccination for West Nile virus when the foal is three to four months of age. This should be followed by booster vaccinations. Unless the vet has concerns about a specific disease or outbreak in your area, the other vaccinations are usually not begun until after the foal is weaned, or around five or six months of age.

Discuss with the vet the best vaccination plan for your horses. Recommendations will vary depending on your area and your specific situation. (See Vaccine Guidelines box in chapter 10.)

If for any reason the mare was not properly vaccinated during pregnancy, the foal's entire immunization program may need to begin prior to weaning, or at three to four months of age.

Deworming

You may be feeding an adequate ration of grain, but if you don't have a plan to manage internal parasites, your horse can still develop nutritional deficiencies. Internal parasites damage the horse's intestinal lining, affecting digestion and the absorption of nutrients. They can also cause diarrhea, blindness, and colic.

Your foal should be on a routine deworming program to control internal parasites, starting

Common Signs of Parasite Infestation

- Soft cough, followed by swallowing (roundworms migrate through the lungs)
- Scruffy coat
- Dense hair along the midline under the belly (may look like a goat's beard)

Make Deworming Easier

If you find it tough to deworm your foal now, imagine how much more difficult it could be when he's older and weighs 1,000 pounds!

The next time the vet visits, ask her for a large (60 cc) plastic syringe, or buy one at your tack and supply store. Make deworming easier on both of you by investing just a few minutes a week in the following desensitization training.

When you are going out to groom the foal, mix up two or three tablespoons of plain applesauce with a little molasses and put the mixture in the syringe. Allow the foal to sniff the syringe and then administer some of the contents in the same way you would a deworming product as described on page 78. Most horses find the mixture tasty and will want more. If you practice this just a few times a month during some of your grooming sessions, the foal will soon associate an oral dose syringe or deworming tube with something positive.

Many medications are administered orally. If and when you have to treat the foal later in life, it will be much easier if he doesn't struggle when you put something into his mouth.

at one to two months. Look for deworming products that specifically state they are safe for young foals, such as fenbendazole (brand names Safeguard and Panacur). You may have already used such a dewormer at foal heat. Read the label carefully, as certain products are not suggested for use until the foal is older. Ask your veterinarian for her advice on deworming products, and follow instructions to the letter.

How to Deworm the Foal

The easiest way to deworm the foal for the first time is in a small, confined area such as the stall. Ask someone to hold the mare, or tie her so she cannot interfere as you handle the foal.

Halter the foal and position him so he is standing against one wall or with his rump in a corner. If you have another person handy, he can cradle the foal with one arm at the foal's chest and another at the hindquarters.

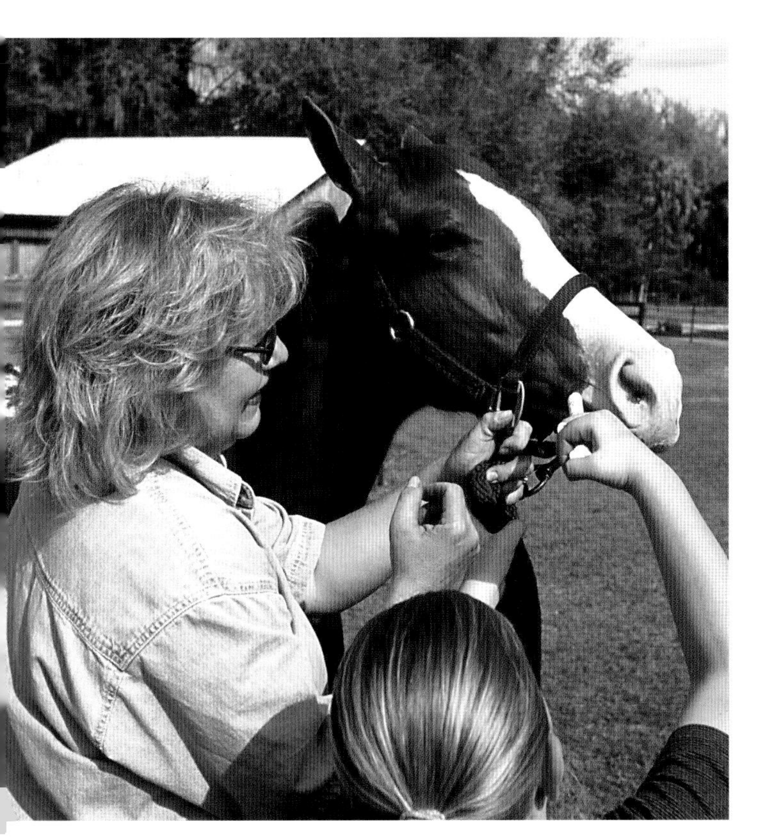

Slide the dewormer plunger into the side of the foal's mouth, not the front.

If the foal has been nursing or eating grain, you or your assistant should hold him quietly and let him stand a few minutes to make sure he swallows anything in his mouth. If any grass, feed, or hay remains in his mouth, he will try to spit it out when you give him the dewormer, and much of the medication will be spat out, as well.

Adjust the plunger on the tube of dewormer so the dose is accurate. Stand to the left or right of the foal but never directly in front of him; if he decides to jump forward, you could be hurt. Place one hand on the bridge of the foal's nose to hold his head steady, and with your other hand slide the end of the deworming tube into the back corner of his mouth where there are no teeth. Don't try to insert the tube from the front of his mouth; he will bite it. Depress the plunger so the medication is deposited into the back of his mouth. Tilt the foal's head upward slightly and keep his mouth closed to encourage him to swallow the deworming medication.

Don't be in a hurry to finish up. If you let go of him immediately after you remove the tube, he will likely lower his head and spit out the medication. And instantly releasing him will reinforce the idea that this is something unpleasant to be gotten away from as soon as possible. Instead, hold on to the foal for a few minutes after giving him the dewormer. Praise and stroke him so he does not consider this a negative experience.

Maintain your foal, along with his dam and any other horses on the premises, on a routine deworming program. On large farms in mild climates and with many horses, they may need to be dewormed every four to six weeks. At the very least, adult horses should be dewormed four times a year; young horses should be dewormed more frequently. Talk with your vet about setting up a regular program to fight parasites.

Warning!

Some people use horse dewormers to treat their dogs. *Never* do this unless specifically advised to by your dog's veterinarian. Too high a dose or the wrong kind of dewormer can easily kill a dog or at the least make him very ill. Stick to medication designed for dogs and leave the equine dewormers to horses.

Hoof Care

Your foal should have his first hoof trimming at about 1 month unless the veterinarian suggests otherwise. Proper trimming will help build a solid foundation for the foal's developing feet and legs. Potential problems may be avoided by paying close attention to the young horse's hoof care. Future soundness can be compromised by neglect or poor trimming practices.

At the first visit, the blacksmith, also referred to as a **farrier,** should watch the foal walk toward and away from him before any trimming is done. He should also watch the foal walk after he has been trimmed. This way he can assess how the foal places his feet when he walks and how the hoof itself comes in contact with the ground. He can also notice any gait peculiarities while the foal is walking.

Most of the time, the blacksmith will be using only a rasp and hoof knife on young foals. Because good balance is the goal of the initial visits, the blacksmith will trim the foot to encourage it to land flat when it contacts the ground. Smoothing and shaping the hoof wall will help it become thicker and more resilient. In young foals, the sole is quite thin and the frog is typically not trimmed much, if at all, for the first few months of trimming.

Put your foal on a routine trimming program in which he is trimmed every four to six weeks. If your foal has specific hoof or limb problems, the vet and the farrier will devise a customized trimming and hoof-care program, and he will likely need to be trimmed more frequently.

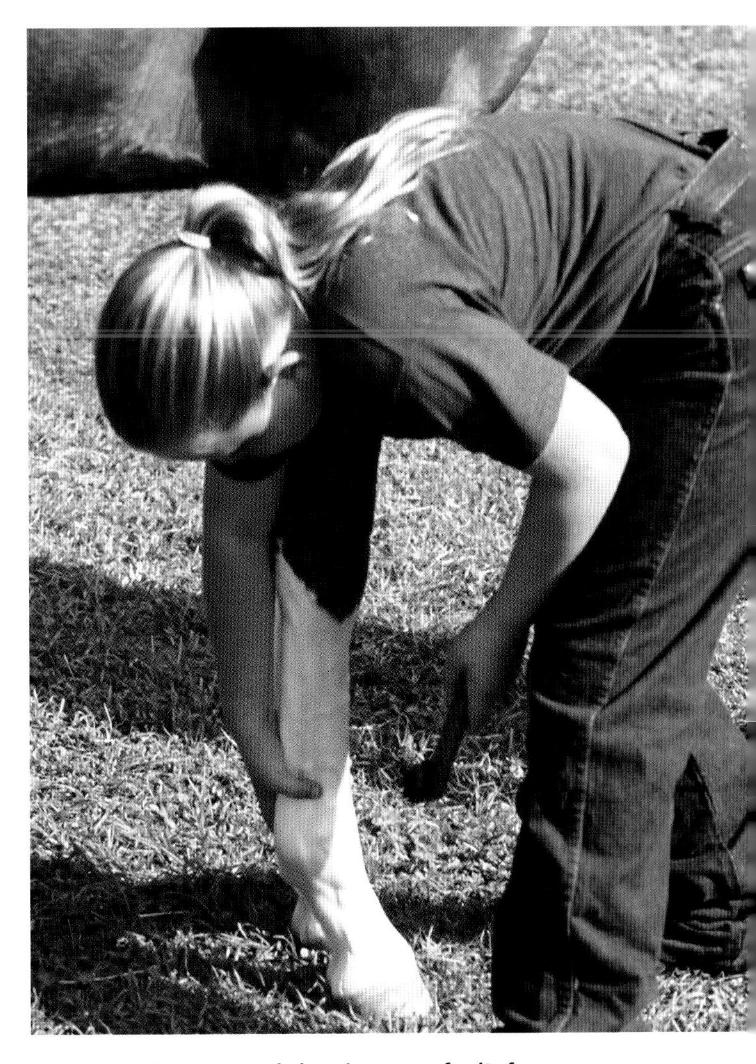

Practice picking up and cleaning your foal's feet regularly so he will mind his manners when the blacksmith comes.

Play It Safe!

Whenever the vet or blacksmith is working on your horse, for safety's sake always stand on the same side of the horse as the other person.

Keep a Photo Record

You may think you will remember every detail about the first months of your foal's life, but don't rely on memory alone. When it comes to important details such as hoof care, a photo record is especially valuable. You should also make notes of any specific comments your blacksmith has at each trimming. (See chapter 12, "Record Keeping.")

Make it a point to take a series of photos after each blacksmith visit for the first several months or even the first year of the foal's life. The foal should be standing still with all four feet flat on the ground. If possible, he should stand square, with all four legs straight underneath him and the front and back legs even with each other.

How Do Horses Age?

You may be familiar with how dogs age as compared to humans, but what about the horse?

In the first year of life, the foal grows rapidly compared to a human child. From birth until 3 years, the horse ages approximately 6.5 years for every human year. In his third year of life, the horse's aging slows to about 5 years for every human year. The 3-year-old horse is the rough equivalent of an 18-year-old human. From 4 years on, the horse ages only about 2.5 years for each human year. A 22-year-old horse is approximately 65 years old in human terms. A horse that lives to the ripe old age of 36 is the equivalent of a 100-year-old person.

All age equivalents in the charts are approximate, and just as with humans, some animals age better than others.

Dog	Human
1 year	15 years
2 years	24 years
4 years	32 years
7 years	45 years
10 years	56 years
15 years	76 years
20 years	98 years

Horse	Human
1 year	6½ years
2 years	13 years
3 years	18 years
4 years	20½ years
10 years	35½ years
17 years	53 years
20 years	60½ years
24 years	70½ years
30 years	85½ years
36 years	100½ years

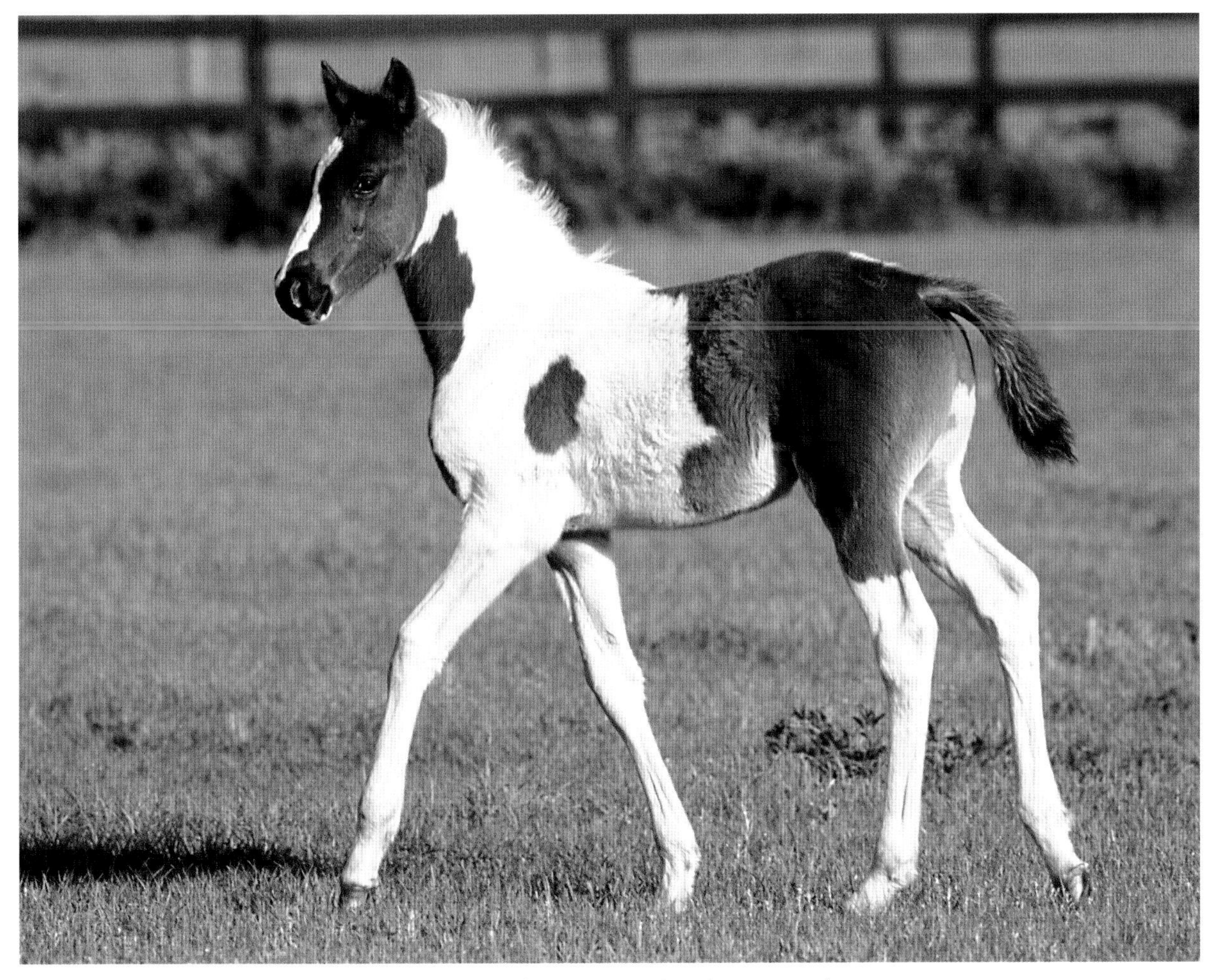

Proper nutrition is critical during your horse's first year to develop strong bones and obtain maximum muscle growth.

Take at least six photos:

- One from the foal's left side
- One from the foal's right side
- One from the front
- One from the rear
- A close-up view of the two front feet, from the knees down, taken from the front
- A view of the two hind feet, from the hocks down, taken from the rear

Label the photos with a date and the foal's name, if there are several foals on the farm. This will make it easy to notice improvements or changes in the foal's hooves and legs as he grows.

8

Four to Six Months

Confidence and Curiosity

That old phrase "growing like a weed" certainly applies to the foal at this age. Not only is he growing physically, but by the age of 4 to 6 months, he is also maturing mentally.

Although still nursing and dependent on his mother to some degree, the foal is gaining confidence and becoming curious about the world around him. If he is kept with other youngsters his age, they will spend a lot of time interacting. It is common to see foals grazing and playing together in a group while their mothers graze or rest nearby. This is a natural process as the foal becomes more independent and prepared for weaning and separation from his dam.

Mare Nutrition

In late lactation, from 4 months until weaning, both the supply and the quality of the mare's milk drop considerably. Feeding the mare a concentrate containing fat and high-quality protein can slow this decline.

Her nutrition requirements won't be as great as during the first three months after foaling. The mare's forage needs will remain similar, but she will not require as much nutrition from concentrates.

Foal Nutrition

By the fourth month of lactation, the mare's milk is providing less than 30 percent of the total energy needed by her foal. Continue making grain or concentrates available (see chapter 7) to ensure that the foal receives the nutrition he needs for growth. He will gradually be eating more concentrate from 4 to 6 months, but keep in mind that the rule is no more than 1 pound of feed per month of age. For example, a 4-month-old foal shouldn't be given more than 4 pounds of concentrate per day.

By providing a quality, balanced commercial ration designed for the growing foal, you can rest assured that he is receiving the correct proportions of protein, energy, calcium, phosphorus, vitamins, and minerals for healthy bone development as he grows and puts on weight.

Contact your veterinarian if you notice any heat, knots, or swelling around the foal's knees or ankles or changes in the angles of the foal's legs. These can be signs of developmental orthopedic disease (DOD) or **epiphysitis** (inflammation of the growth plates of bones). The foal's diet may need to be adjusted, but do not make changes without discussing this with your vet. Forage, ration, total energy intake, and exercise are all components of DOD and of epiphysitis, and the vet can explain changes you need to make in any or all of these.

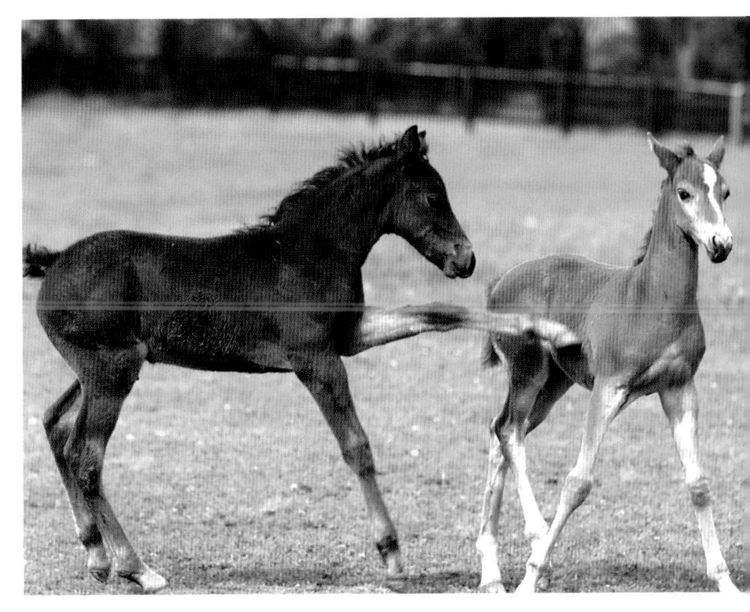
Social interaction is an important part of the foal's life.

Health Care from Four to Six Months

Your foal may or may not need to start an immunization program at this time, so discuss this with your vet. Other health care issues, such as deworming and hoof care, should continue routinely.

Vaccinations

At about 4 months of age, the foal may need certain vaccinations, depending on your geographic region. If the mare was properly vaccinated during pregnancy, the foal won't need most vaccines until after weaning, at 5 to 6 months. Be sure to talk with your veterinarian about your horse's specific immunization needs.

Deworming

Continue the established deworming program, making sure to use only products approved for your foal's age and weight. Depending on the region and where your horses are stabled, you may need to deworm as frequently as every 30 days. For example, if your mare and foal are pastured with a group of mares and foals, deworm them more frequently than if there were no other horses sharing their pasture. If left untreated, parasites can cause permanent damage to the young horse, so make it a point to maintain a parasite-prevention routine.

Mare Nutrition during Late Lactation

Forage: 1–2% of mare's body weight
Concentrate: 0.5–1.5% of mare's body weight
Total daily intake: 2–2.5% of mare's body weight

Example: (adjust to your specific mare's weight and needs)

- 1,000-pound mare × 1 to 2% of body weight in forage = 10 to 20 pounds forage (1 to 2 pounds forage per 100 pounds body weight)
- 1,000-pound mare × 0.5 to 1.5% concentrate = 5 to 15 pounds concentrate (0.5 to 1.5 pounds concentrate per 100 pounds body weight)

Total feed ration: approximately 20–25 pounds/day

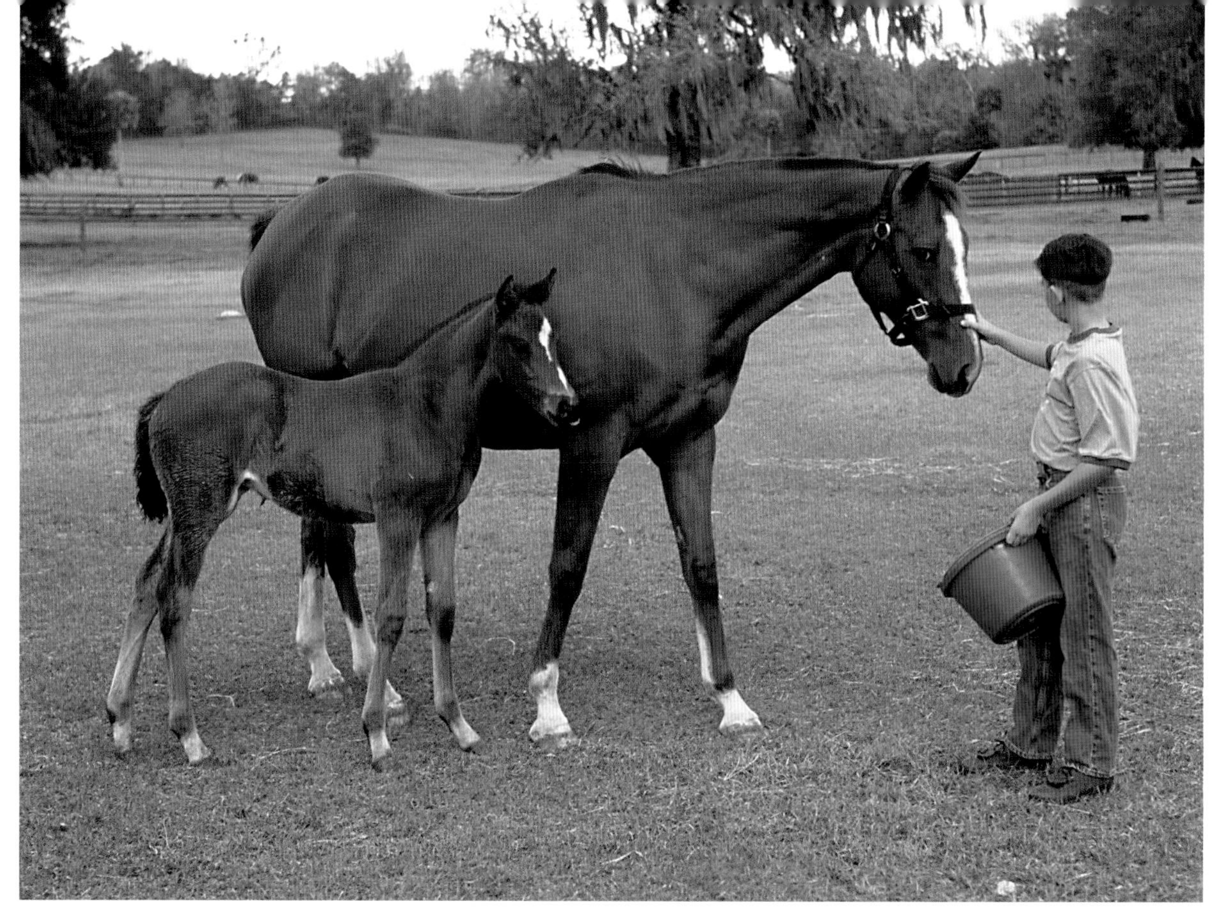

Foals need a feed designed specifically for them to ensure that they receive the necessary nutrients.

Tapeworms may not present a problem until your foal is older, but studies have shown that tapeworm infestation is a leading cause of colic in horses. Not all dewormers are effective against tapeworms, so read the label or ask your vet if you aren't sure what to use. Add dewormer that targets tapeworms to your parasite-prevention program at least twice a year — or more frequently if your vet advises. She will tell you when to start deworming the young horse for tapeworms.

Hoof Care

Continue with the foal's established hoof-care and trimming program, following the recommendations of the blacksmith and veterinarian.

Contrary to what some horse owners think, most horses do not need hoof dressing on a regular basis. Many people like the way the hoof dressing or ointment looks, but applying

Feeding Snacks

It's natural to want to give your horses snacks, but don't make this a habit every time you work with them. If you do, they will learn to expect it and may start invading your space, trying to locate the treat. Colts, especially, can become nippy if they think you always have a snack.

When you do give a treat, it's best to offer it at the end of a grooming or training session. To discourage a horse from nibbling at your clothes or hands, put the snack in the feed bucket instead of feeding it by hand.

it when it is not required can actually weaken a horse's feet, as they become overly hydrated. Some hoof-care products will also attract dirt and fecal matter, which can cause problems if there are cracks in the hoof. Paradoxically, they can even dry out the hoof by packing too much dirt on the outer surface and causing cracks.

Certain hoof problems are genetic; others are related to the environment and nutrition. The bottom line is to apply hoof-care products only when necessary. Your blacksmith can advise you on specific products if a horse needs them.

Exercise

In order for your foal to develop properly, plenty of exercise is essential. Veterinarians recommend that foals not be confined for more than ten hours a day unless there is a medical reason. Some respiratory infections can also be avoided if foals spend most of their time outdoors.

At this age, the foal doesn't need forced exercise, such as round-pen work, which can put stress on young joints and limbs. Simply being turned out with his mother in a pasture of at least an acre will give the foal room to run and play.

Foals and their mothers should be turned out as much as possible. In many areas, weather permitting, they can be outdoors around the clock. During the warm months, you may want to bring them inside only for feeding and handling. If you leave horses outside, ensure that adequate shade, shelter, and water are available at all times.

If you feed outside, spend at least a short period each day closely observing mare and foal so you will notice any changes in appetite, appearance, or attitude. And don't forget that daily handling, even for just a few minutes, will go a long way toward making your foal easier to work with as he grows.

Beyond Routine Grooming

Sooner or later, you'll have to do more than just brush your foal and pick out his feet. This is a great age to introduce bathing and clipping, so he becomes accustomed to these routines.

Bathing Your Foal

By the time the foal is several months old, he will probably have had many "natural baths", in the rain. But being sprayed by a long, snake-like hose may create fear, so you want to make his first official bath a pleasant experience.

If the mare likes a bath, use her as a "model" when you introduce the foal to bathing. (If she is finicky or nervous about bathing, don't use this method, as her anxiety can transfer to the foal, who will then start to think a bath isn't such a good idea after all.) Halter the mare and have someone hold her with a lead rope in the paddock or pen near the fence. Leave the foal loose in the paddock with her while you wash the mare with the hose. Soap is optional this time; the idea is to accustom the foal to the sights and sounds of bathing before he is the one being washed.

Rub It In!

Regular, daily massage of the **coronary band,** the area at the top of the hoof where the hair meets the hoof, will stimulate growth.

Some veterinarians and blacksmiths believe that both hoof quality and growth can be increased by rubbing the coronary band with a dry, stiff toothbrush or hoof brush 2 minutes per day per hoof.

Your Foal's First Bath

If you live where the summers are hot, give your foal his first "official" bath on a sunny day. Otherwise, choose a mild day and use warm water in a bucket instead of a hose. Plan to give this first bath midday or early afternoon so he has plenty of time to dry off before the temperature drops later in the day.

Soap isn't necessary for the first bath, but you will want to have some on hand for later baths. You can use horse shampoo, available at any tack and supply store, or a mild human shampoo.

If the foal is not yet weaned, keep the mare close by to reassure him that all is well. If the mare stands quietly when tied, you can tie her near the bathing area, or have someone hold her. Don't leave her loose, however; if she decides to walk away when you're in the middle of washing the foal, he may become alarmed and try to bolt after her.

1. Have an assistant hold the foal for the first bath rather than tying him. Once the foal is older and has learned to stand tied and is familiar with being bathed, use a quick-release knot to tie him.

2. Introduce the foal to water coming out of the hose by running it on his lower legs first, not on his body. Don't use a harsh spray, and make sure the water isn't too hot or too cold. Let the water run gently in a low stream. Speak calmly and reassuringly throughout the bathing session, praising the foal and rewarding him with strokes and rubs when he stands still. If you are using warm water in a bucket instead of a hose, use a sponge to soak up the water and then squeeze it over the foal's legs.

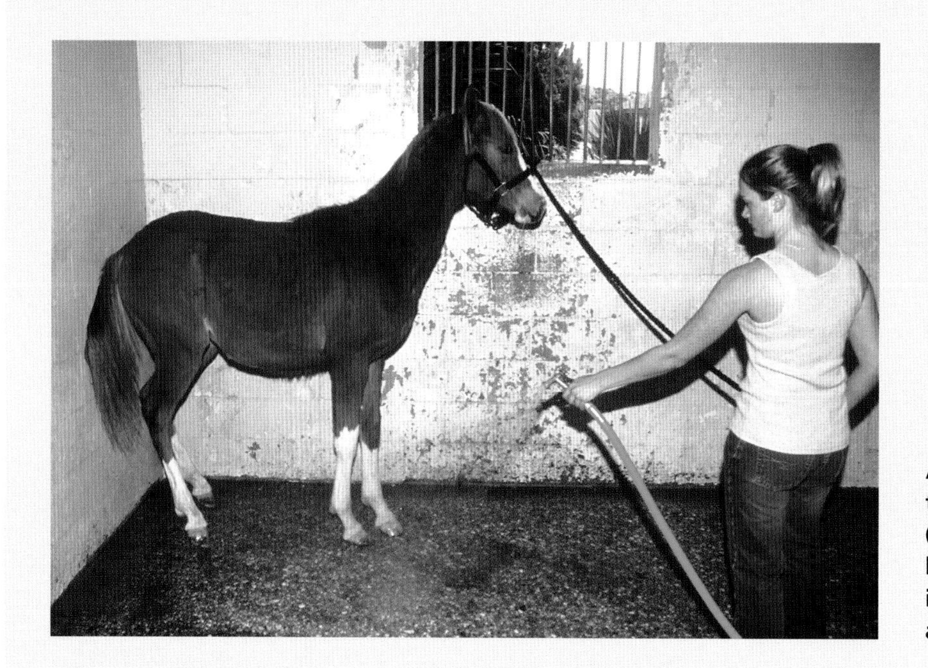

Always start by wetting the feet and legs (step 2). Note that the horse in these photos is a weanling and has already learned to tie.

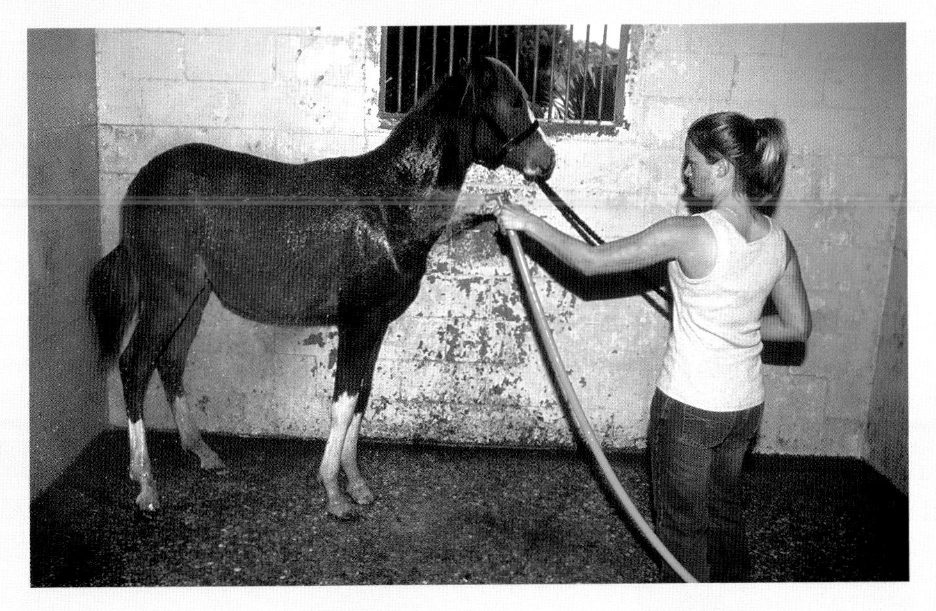

Once the foal accepts water on his legs, work up to spraying his body, starting with the shoulders and front end (step 3).

If you like, use a soft brush during the bath (step 5). The foal is familiar with this from his grooming sessions.

3. It may take several minutes for the foal to begin to accept the water streaming down his legs. Once he does, slowly move the water up to his chest area. Don't wet the sensitive belly or flanks at first. Wet his chest, shoulders, and then lower neck. If he starts to get nervous, go back to running the water on an area he has already accepted, such as down his legs.

4. Slowly move the hose until the water is running across the foal's back. After he accepts this, you can wet his rump and flanks. Don't wet his head at all for the first bath.

(continued on next page)

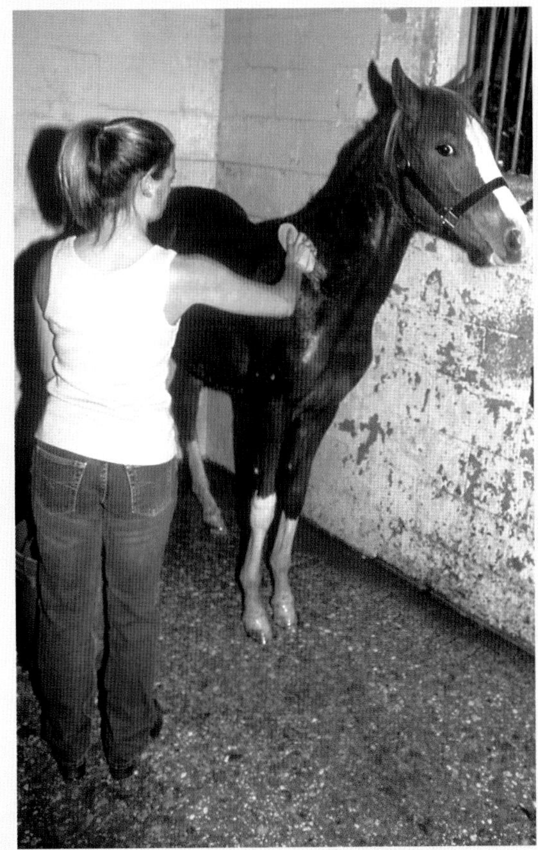

Your Foal's First Bath *(continued)*

5. Use a rubber currycomb or soft brush on his body with one hand while you continue to run the water on him. Because you have been grooming the foal regularly, he will be accustomed to this, which may help him settle down and even enjoy the first bath.

6. Turn off the hose and rub the foal's body gently with a sweat scraper or the edge of your hand to remove excess water. Never use a scraper on a horse's legs; it may be uncomfortable or irritating.

7. Spend a few minutes after bathing to brush the foal lightly or rub a towel over his body. These familiar actions from past grooming sessions will reinforce that the bathing ritual is a good experience.

8. In later bathing sessions, you can wash the foal's face. Use a sponge or washcloth dipped in water rather than spraying his face with a hose. He is accustomed to having his face brushed while grooming, so the sponge or cloth won't be frightening, and you won't risk getting water in his ears.

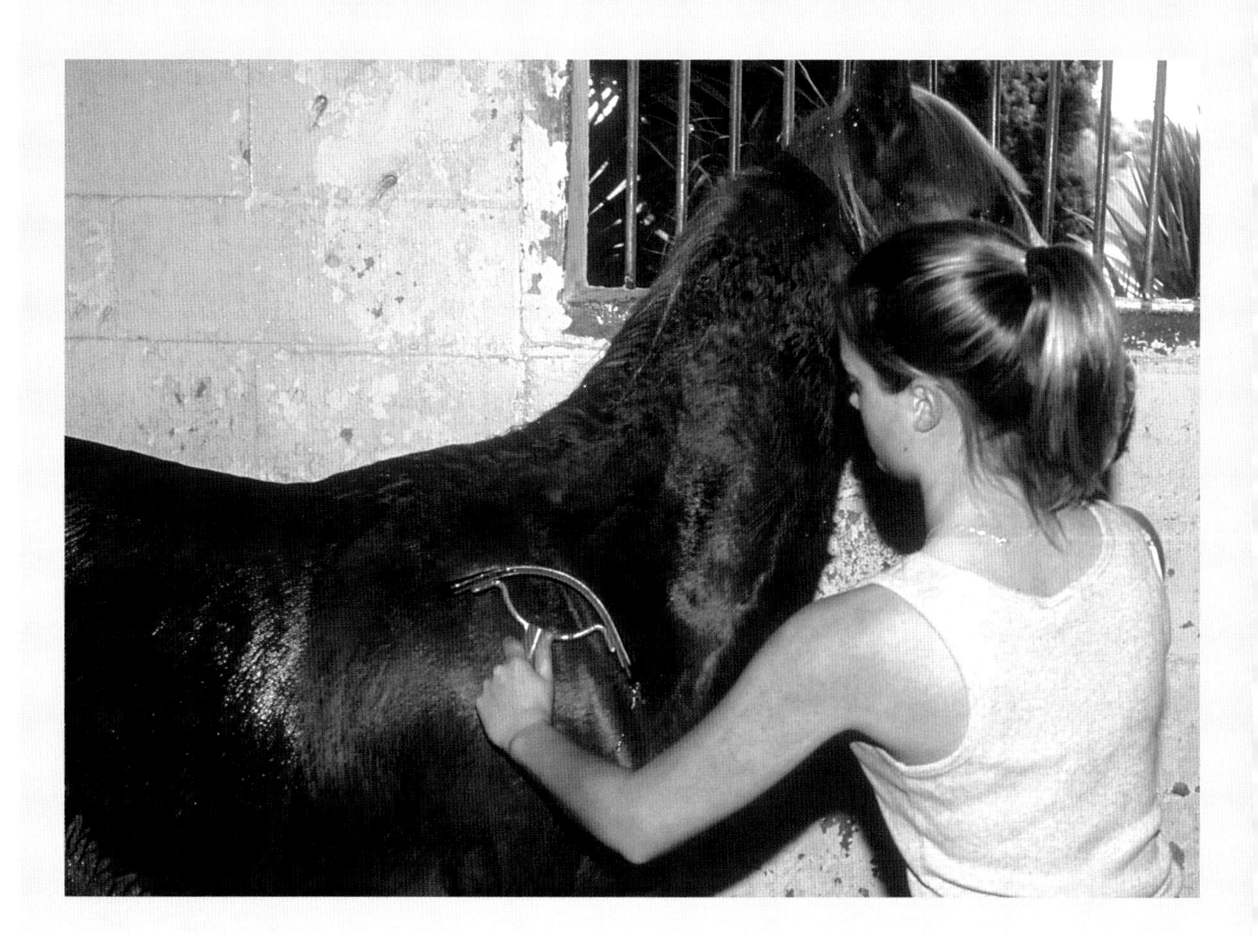

Tips for Success

This first bath shouldn't last longer than necessary. The idea is not to clean the foal as much as it is to get him to peacefully accept being bathed. Your goal is to make the experience relaxing and pleasant. Do everything you can to make bathing a positive memory.

If you have been handling the foal routinely over the past months and act quietly and calmly, he should accept this first bath within a few minutes. If for some reason he doesn't relax and accept the experience, don't feel you have to wet his entire body now. Once the foal learns to stand quietly for a bath when he is young, you will never face the challenge of trying to wash an upset adult horse.

After your foal has had a few water baths and is comfortable, you can start using shampoo. You just want to be sure he has accepted the routine so you know he will stand to be rinsed well.

Dilute the shampoo by pouring some into a bucket with water. Apply it with a sponge once the foal's body is completely wet. For dirty spots, pour shampoo directly onto a rubber currycomb, brush, or sponge and rub the foal's body with it. In either case, be sure to rinse all of the shampoo off the body — remembering the belly and legs — when you are finished.

Gently remove excess water with the sweat scraper after you are finished washing the foal (step 6).

The foal will probably want to investigate what is going on. Don't intentionally spray him with water, as this may frighten him, but if he gets splashed while you're washing the mare, that's fine. Because he's loose, he has the option of walking off if he doesn't want any part of it. If the mare is calm and enjoying her bath, however, the foal will become naturally curious and want to join in the activity.

Both handlers need to be alert and not have their backs to the foal in case he decides to buck or run around the mare.

Clipping

You may intend to show your foal after he is weaned. In that case, it's a good idea to get him used to being clipped at an early age.

Before you actually do any clipping, turn on the electric clippers during a couple of grooming sessions to accustom the foal to their vibration and sound. Rub them against the foal's body while they are running, with the blade side turned away from the hair.

At this stage, you don't have to clip more than just his **fetlocks,** or ankles, and touch up any long hairs under the jaw. It isn't necessary to clip your foal's ears or muzzle; the ears especially benefit from their fuzzy protection against dust, flies, and other insects.

If you want to, clip a short **bridle path,** the part of the horse's mane just behind his ears. This will leave a flat area on which the halter can rest. Arabians traditionally have a longer bridle path than that of other breeds, but for most horses, especially foals, a short bridle path of just an inch or two is plenty. For a general measurement, take the horse's ear and gently press it back flat on his neck. Don't clip farther back than where the tip of the ear lies.

In regions where summers are hot, some owners do a partial clip on their foals if the babies have not shed their winter coats by the time hot weather arrives. Typically, the chest

Clipping

Have someone hold the foal while you use the clippers. The horse's hair should be clean and dry before any clipping. *Never try to clip a wet or damp horse!*

For trimming the bridle path, jaw, and fetlocks, use #10 clipper blades. Oil and lubricate the clippers as necessary, according to the manufacturer's recommendations.

Use two hands when clipping: one to operate the clippers and the other to rest on the horse. It is always good to have a second point of physical contact with the foal. When you are clipping the bridle path, rest your free hand reassuringly on the bridge of the horse's nose to steady him as you clip. When you are trimming hair on the legs and fetlocks, rest your free hand on the same leg you are working on.

When using electric clippers, be aware of the cord at all times. Keep it away from the foal's teeth and out from under his feet. Horses have been electrocuted by biting into cords. Because foals, like human babies, like to put everything in their mouths, a set of cordless rechargeable clippers is a good alternative to electric clippers. Tack stores and catalogs offer a variety of clippers.

Thoroughly brush or wipe a damp sponge over the area you have clipped to remove any loose hair.

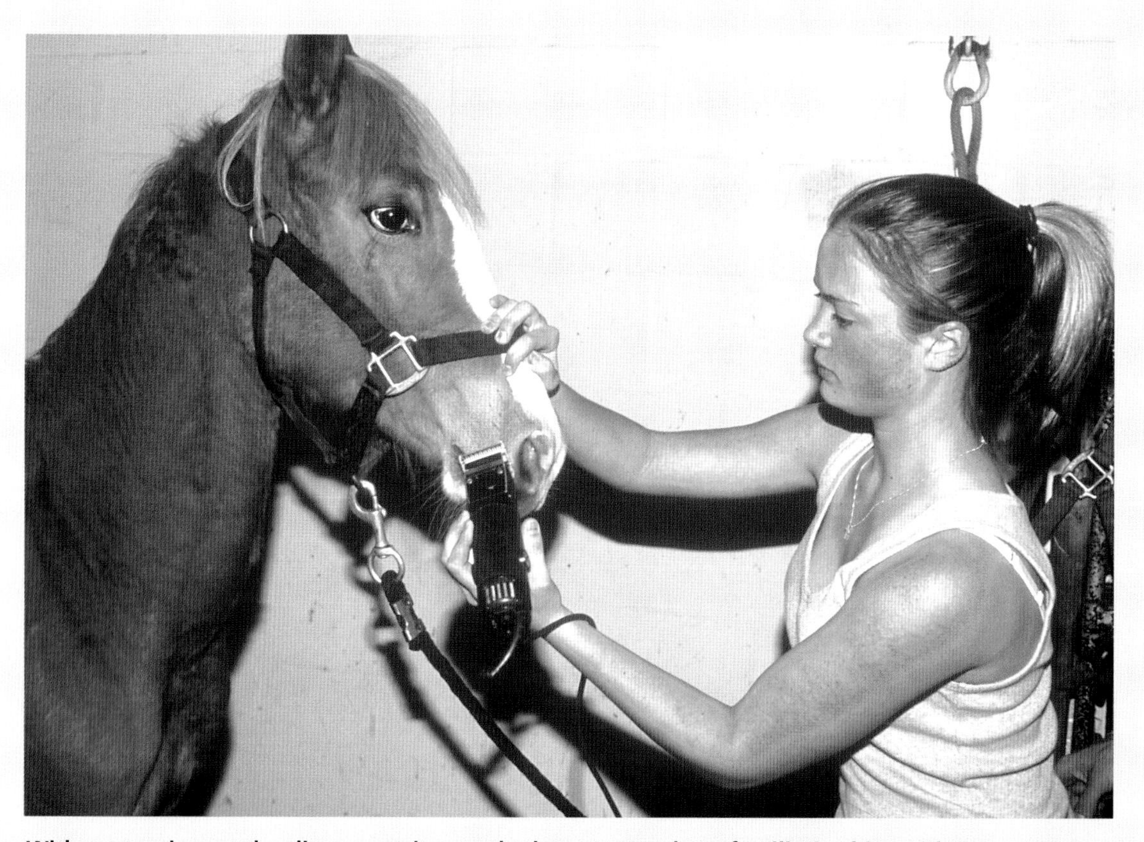

Without turning on the clipper, run it over the horse's muzzle to familiarize him with it.

and sides from about the middle of the **barrel** (the horse's midsection) and back to the flanks are clipped close. These are the areas where the horse tends to sweat the most. Clipping the hair shorter here will help keep the horse cooler. Eventually, the foal will shed out completely and there will be no clip line.

Trailer Loading

At some point in your foal's life, he will have to travel in a horse trailer or van. The earlier he becomes familiar with loading and is comfortable inside a trailer, the easier it will be for everyone when he is older.

It is best to teach your foal to load when you don't actually need to go anywhere. That way you can relax during the learning process without worrying about arriving on time. Later, when you need to trailer to a show, a club event, or the veterinarian, your horse will already load easily.

Veterinarians see many injuries that are the result of horses getting hurt in trailers, often while loading or unloading. If you can make the introduction to the trailer a calm and pleasant one, the foal will have no reason to think of the trailer as a scary, dangerous place.

Horses become afraid when they think they will be hurt or unable to flee from danger. If your horse is afraid of the trailer because it is a new experience for him, the last thing you want to do is make him load into it. Using force will simply strengthen his fear that the trailer is a bad place to be, and he will be even more reluctant to load the next time.

It is possible to override an established fear and eventually train a balky horse to load, but the best method is simply not to create bad habits from the beginning. Always keep in mind that the foal never forgets first experiences.

Although the trailer-loading lesson is included in this chapter, you do not have to wait until the foal is four to six months old to introduce him to loading. Foals as young as a month old can learn to load safely; it is often even easier to teach a younger foal to load.

End on the Positive!

Any time you are working with a horse, you must end the session on a positive note, no matter what you are trying to teach the animal and how little you accomplish. For example, if you're trying to give the foal his first bath and he doesn't want any part of it, you have to find something he knows and accepts before you end the session.

If he is afraid of the hose, turn down the water to just a trickle. If he wants to sniff the hose, let him. Another option is to put lukewarm water in a bucket and use a sponge to first wet his legs before reintroducing water from the hose. You may want to end by giving the foal a short grooming session in the same place you give the bath.

Think of "building blocks" whenever you want to introduce something to a horse, no matter his age. Start with something the horse knows and understands, begin teaching the new experience, and always end with something the horse is familiar with and does well. You can always build on a positive session, but if you stop when things aren't going well, you can be sure the foal will remember.

Loading into a Trailer

To teach your foal to load safely and easily, you'll need to take safety precautions before starting. Most important is to provide safe footing and a closed-in area where the foal can be contained, because he will be left loose in the first lessons.

Preparation

Back up the truck and horse trailer to an area that can be closed in, such as the aisle of a barn or the gateway of a pen or small paddock. Shut the doors on the other end of the barn or close any gates in the pen. The only exit should lead into the trailer. Remove buckets, feed tubs, and any other equipment in the vicinity.

It may be easier on the foal if the trailer has a ramp, but this is not necessary. If you have a step-up trailer, try to park it such that the distance from the ground to the trailer floor is as short as possible.

A horse does not have the same depth perception as a human has. He cannot tell if a puddle is just inches deep or 10 feet deep. To him, a dark spot on the ground or a shadow across the trail looks like a black hole. Similarly, the dark interior of a trailer may appear to be a long tunnel or dark cave, and for the horse, nothing friendly can be expected to live in a cave!

To illuminate the trailer interior, fully open the back doors to the trailer and open any windows. If there is an escape door, keep it closed. This door tends to be too small for an adult horse to fit through, but a foal might manage to escape that way or, worse, become stuck in it.

If possible, remove the divider in the trailer. Our loading lesson is easier if the trailer is large enough that you can turn the horses around as you walk out, rather than having to back them out. There should be nonslip rubber mats on the trailer floor and, if the trailer has one, on the ramp.

First Lesson

For the initial lesson, halter the foal but do not use a lead rope. Leave him loose; he won't be able to go anywhere, as he's in an enclosed area.

You will need two people for this lesson: one to handle the mare and the other to follow the foal.

1. With a halter and lead rope on the mare, walk her up to the trailer. Allow her to sniff the ramp if she wants, then walk her into the trailer. Hold her and let her stand quietly in the trailer.

2. The foal will approach the trailer and may walk right in after his mother or stand there looking in. If he doesn't walk in within a few minutes, stand a few feet behind him so that your presence encourages him to move forward. Never hurry or force the foal inside. Most foals will walk into the trailer in a very short time. After all, they have no reason to fear the trailer, and their mom is inside.

(continued on next page)

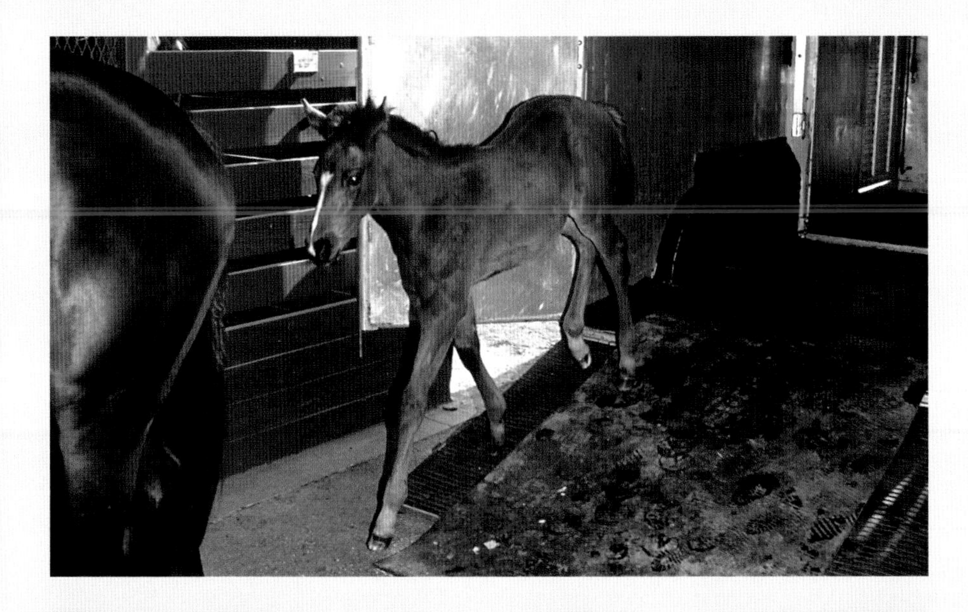

Walk the mare in first and allow the foal to follow (steps 1 and 2).

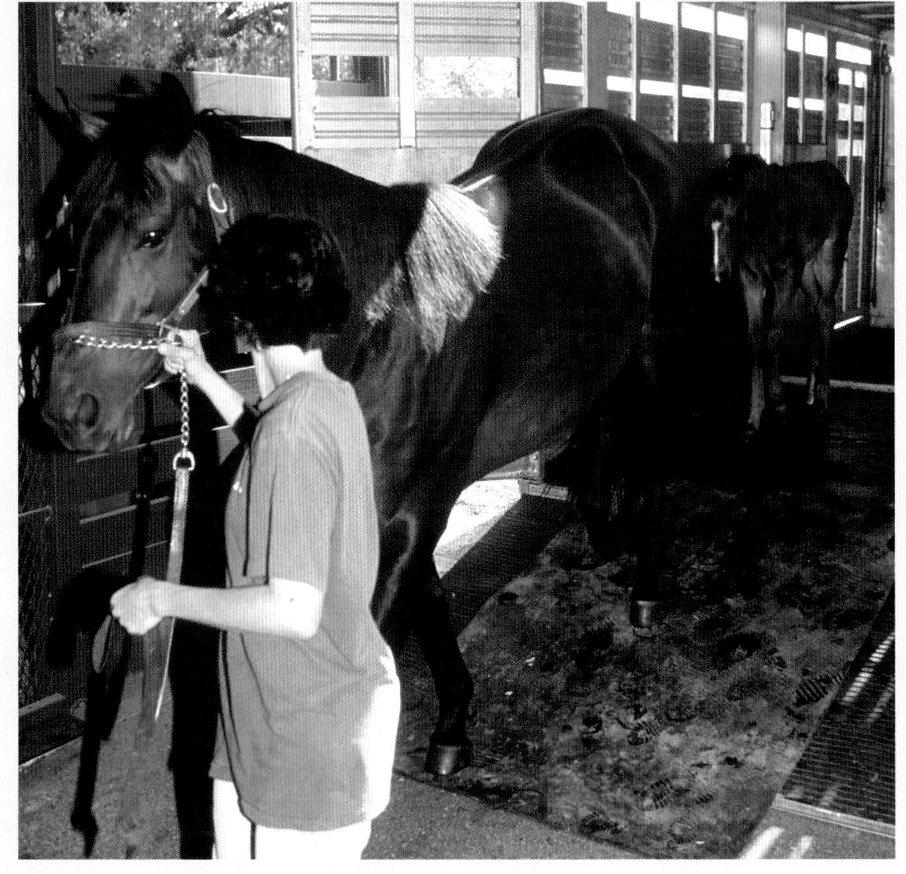

After standing in the trailer for a few minutes, walk the mare out, allowing the foal to follow (step 3).

3. Let both of them stand in the trailer for a minute or two, then walk the mare out slowly and allow the foal to follow.

4. Walk the mare around the pen once or twice, or down the barn aisle. Return to the trailer and repeat the loading exercise. At this point, it is not necessary to close the trailer doors.

5. After they stand in the trailer for a few minutes, walk the horses out. Catch the foal for rubs and praise. Then turn mare and foal back out to pasture or into their stall. Treating them to a little grain now will seal the experience as a positive one.

6. Practice loading once or twice a week.

Next Steps

After the foal has quietly followed his mother into the trailer several times, attach a lead rope to his halter and use a butt rope for encouragement the first few solo times. Every step will be the same as the initial lesson except that someone will actually lead the foal instead of letting him follow the mare while loose.

Once the foal is loading well and seems comfortable in the trailer next to his dam, shut the doors and let the mare and foal stand for a few minutes before unloading. It isn't actually necessary to move the trailer

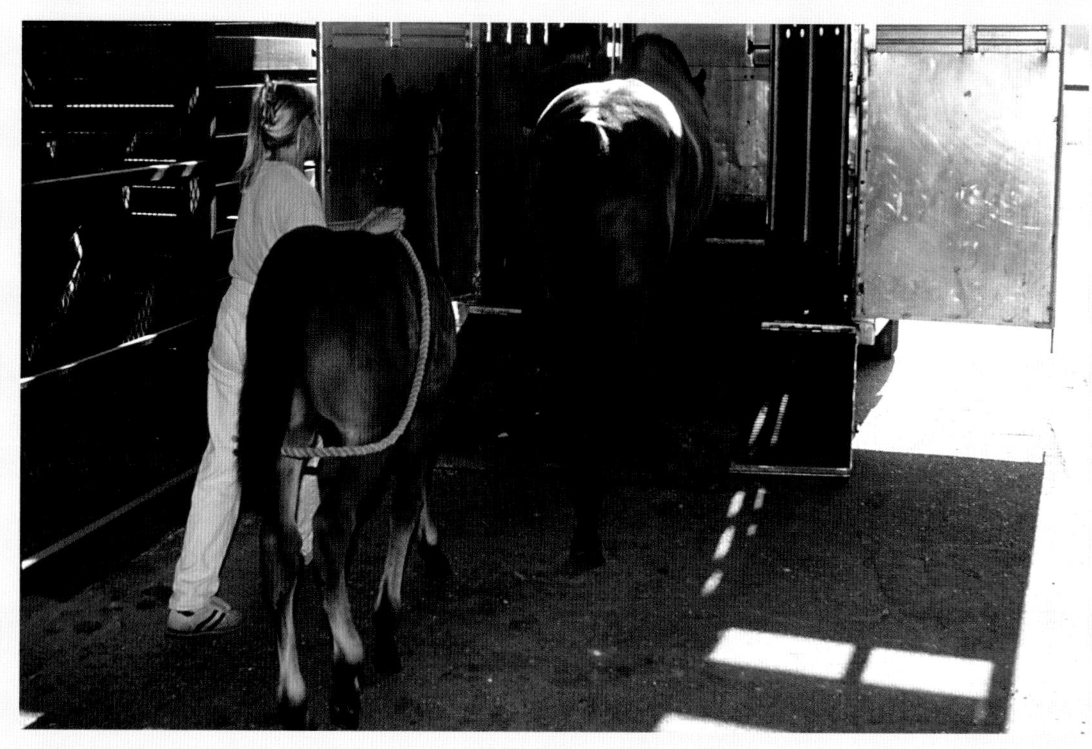

Once the foal can load and unload on his own, start leading him behind the mare. Use a butt rope for encouragement if needed.

with the horses inside, although you can take them for a 5- or 10-minute ride. Here are two important safety reminders:

- Do not have a person stay with the horses in the trailer while it is moving, even on a short trip.
- Never tie a foal in the trailer. Let mare and foal travel loose so they can balance and reposition themselves over rough spots in the road to lessen the possibility of injury.

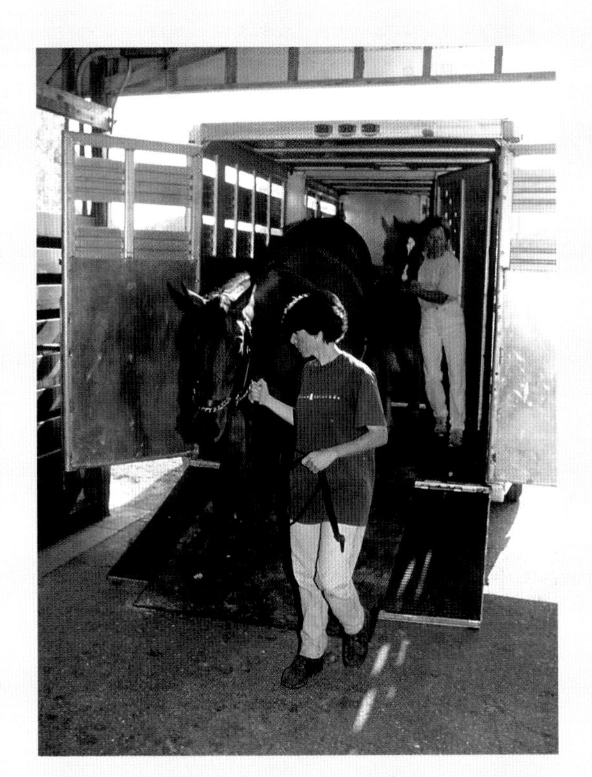

Practice loading when the foal is young, and it will be easy to load him once he is older.

The loading lesson is based on the fact that your mare will load into a trailer quietly and willingly. If she won't, she can't be a good example to the foal and he may pick up her bad habits about loading. A young horse will readily copy the behavior of his mother or another older horse, good or bad. Work with the mare so that she learns to load well, but in the meantime, for safety's sake, you may need to wait until the foal is weaned before proceeding with his lessons. Then you can teach him to load by using another quiet, well-behaved horse as an example.

Just How Smart Are Horses, Anyway?

If you've ever been around someone trying to convince a horse to do something he doesn't want to do, you've probably heard this comment: "Horses are so stupid!"

The fact is that horses simply think differently from humans. Because the horse is a born prey animal, his brain is wired to *run first, think later!* Everything about the horse is designed for fast movement. His highly attuned senses enable him to detect possible danger, and when signaled, his instinct tells him to flee in a hurry.

In the wild, horses have to rapidly evaluate an unfamiliar object and decide if it's something dangerous (a stalking mountain lion) or something they can safely ignore (a branch creaking in the wind). To a horse, the response to every experience is basically *flee* or *ignore.*

You may see a piece of white paper blowing across the barnyard and barely register it; it's nothing. To the horse, however, this is an unfamiliar movement in a place where it is not supposed to be, and that means possible danger.

Because he is a curious creature, you will often see a horse approach a "spooky" object to investigate. He may suddenly turn and run or he will stand his ground once he realizes the object isn't going to get him. Even if he decides the plastic bag blowing across the field isn't deadly, you can be sure he's still poised to flee at any moment.

Horses have poor color vision and see mainly black, white, and pastel-like colors. Black objects and white ones are most visible to the horse, even more than colors such as bright red. This explains why a big black rock along the trail can be considered dangerous.

To anticipate a flight reaction, you have to think like a horse instead of expecting your horse to think like a human. If you are riding down an unfamiliar trail and come across a large dark rock at the base of a tree, you register it visually and immediately categorize it as harmless. Your horse, however, cannot come to the same reasonable conclusion. He simply considers the rock as it appears at first glance, and to him it may resemble a predator crouching by the tree.

Because horses do not reason the same way that humans reason, some people make the mistake of thinking they are stupid. Horses learn very quickly, however, and have an exceptional memory, so in this regard they are highly intelligent. If you can begin to look at the world around you the way a horse does and understand how he experiences it, you will make great strides in handling and working with your equine companion.

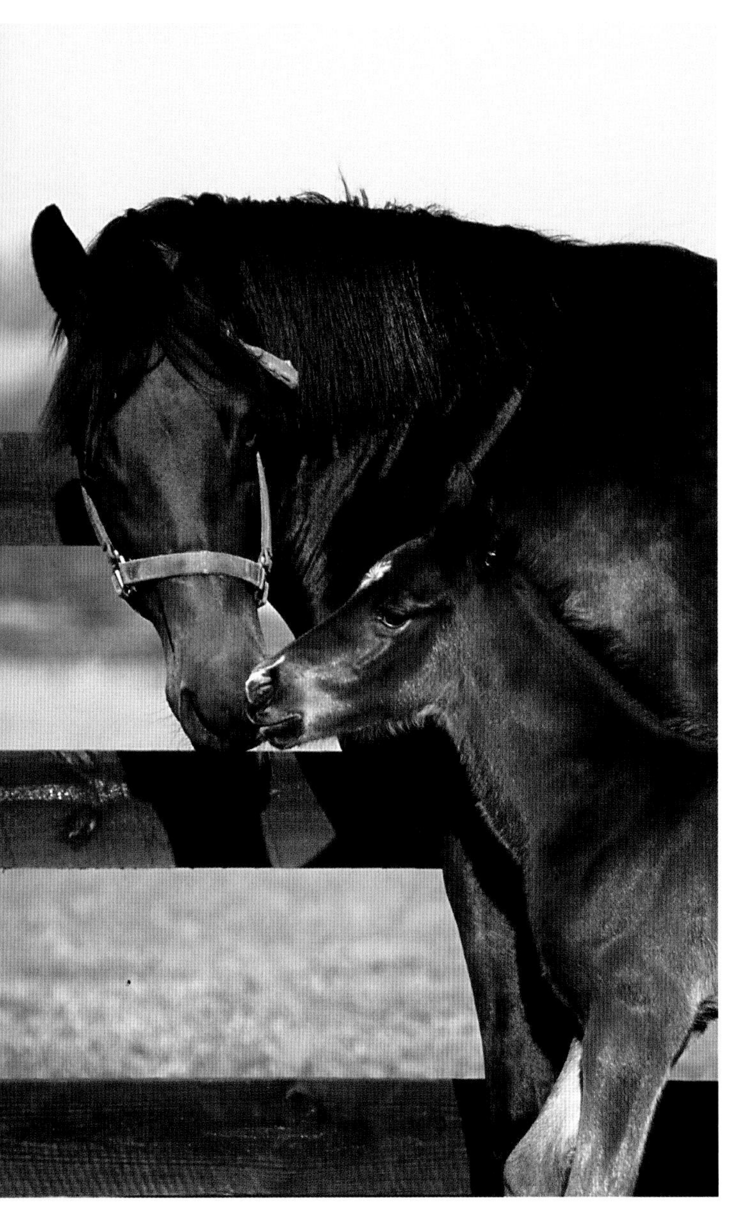

From his very earliest days, the foal's natural instinct is to flee when faced with something alarming or uncertain.

9

Weaning Time

Farewell to Mom

Your foal has traveled a long way since those first wobbly steps. By the time he is 4 to 6 months old, he's a confident, independent young horse who no longer needs his mother. By about 5 months, the foal has learned the social lessons he needs from the dam and it's time to think about **weaning** — that is, permanently separating the foal and his mother.

Mare and foal usually adjust quickly to separation if weaning is done wisely and with common sense. If both mare and foal have at least one other buddy when they are separated, it will be much less stressful on each of them.

When to Wean

In the wild, a mare delivers her foal and is usually bred back by the stallion after she comes into heat while still nursing. As her pregnancy progresses over the months, she will gradually wean her foal. At this point, young horses take different paths according to whether they are male or female. Fillies stay with the herd unless another stallion "steals" them away. Colts will eventually be driven away by the herd stallion as they grow older.

With domesticated horses, owners have to play a role in the process of weaning. Yes, it is possible to leave a foal with his dam indefinitely, and some owners have done this, but there are a number of drawbacks. Riding or showing the mare is quite difficult if her foal is still nursing. If she is bred back again and pregnant with next year's foal, it is natural for her to distance herself, both physically and emotionally, from her current foal. Weaning the foal at an appropriate age also allows you to do lots more activities with the foal and to continue building a strong partnership with him.

When it comes to weaning, the foal's exact age is actually less important than his physical, mental, and social development. You can't just circle a date on the calendar with the plan to wean on the foal's 5-month birthday.

The foal needs to be physically and mentally ready for permanent separation from his dam. He will indicate this by socializing more with his peers and hanging around his mother less. If the mare and foal are the only horses in the field, it is normal for them to seek each other's company, but you will notice the foal ranging farther from his mother and becoming more independent. He will no doubt run to her if he is startled or afraid, but he won't stick close to her side, as he did when he was younger.

The mare's condition is also a factor in weaning. Some mares lose weight and condition the longer they nurse their foals. This may be the case with an older mare or a **hard keeper,** a horse that is tough to keep weight on. When a mare's physical condition is affected by the demands of caring for her foal, you may need to wean earlier than usual. Veterinarians usually recommend waiting until the foal is at least 3 months old. Talk with the vet about early weaning if your mare continues to lose weight or looks "poor," even with an increased feed ration.

When Not to Wean

Do not wean when there are other stress factors. For example, don't combine weaning with a blacksmith or vet visit, or when the horses are being vaccinated or dewormed. Don't wean when new horses are being introduced to the group. If you have to move horses to another pasture or other location, allow them to settle in for at least a week before weaning.

Signs Your Foal Is Ready for Weaning

- Is at least 3 months of age, preferably between 4 and 6 months old
- Routinely eats own ration with a good appetite
- Exhibits good overall physical health
- Grows and develops normally
- Has a normal attitude that is bright and alert
- Shows consistent independence from dam
- Interacts socially with other foals
- Is comfortable being handled, led, and groomed
- Is not under stress from other factors, such as weather
- Enrolled in established blacksmith, deworming, and vaccination programs

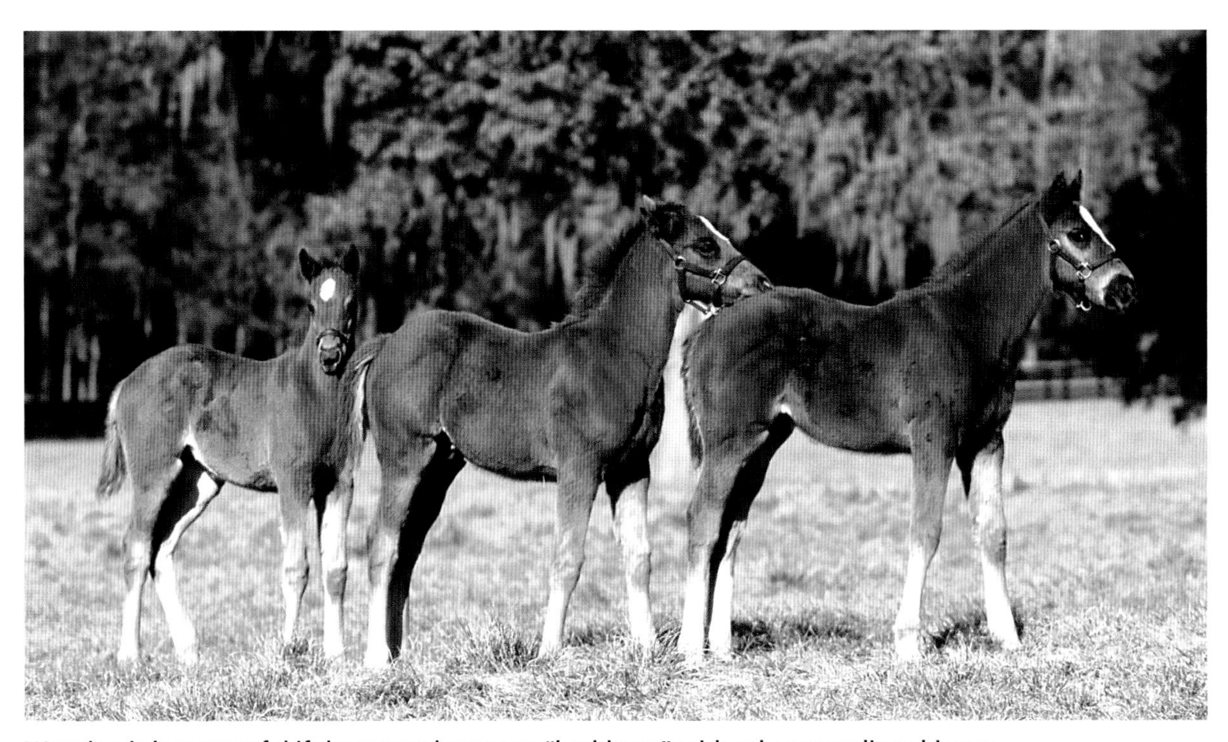

Weaning is less stressful if the young horse can "buddy up" with other weanlings his age.

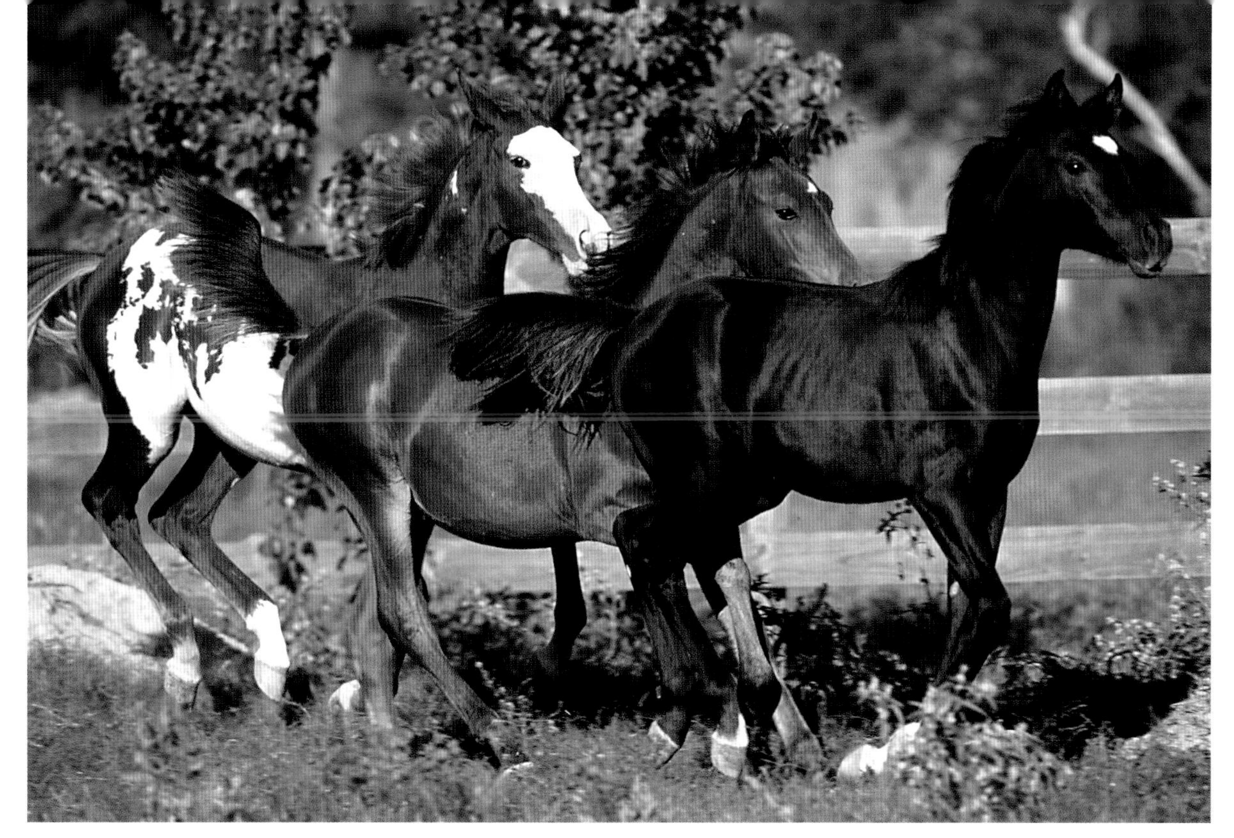

These weanling colts no longer need their dams, but because they are herd animals they will form close social bonds with one another.

Weather can be stressful on horses, particularly during the heat of summer, so avoid weaning on hot, hazy, humid days.

Weaning when either mare or foal is sick or has recently been ill is asking for trouble. Both mare and foal should be in top health at the time of separation.

Methods of Weaning

There are several ways to wean the foal from his dam. The method you choose will depend on your stable/farm arrangement, preference, and the horses themselves. Experts always recommend leaving the foal in familiar surroundings, both for safety and for the foal's comfort level, and relocating the mare.

Gradual weaning begins with separating mare and foal at feeding time by putting them in stalls or pens next to each other. After they have finished eating, they are put back together. The time apart is gradually increased over a period of one to two weeks. Once the foal seems comfortable with the separation, the mare is moved to a location where she can't hear or see her foal. Try to turn out the foal with other new weanlings or a patient "babysitter," such as a docile old pony, friendly burro, or goat.

Studies have shown that group pasture weaning is the least stressful for all concerned. In this method, several mares and foals have been pastured together. As the foals approach weaning time, one or two mares are removed every week to 10 days, taking the dams of the oldest, most independent foals first. These mares are then pastured where they cannot hear or see their foals.

The mares soon settle down because they are with their friends, and their newly weaned foals stay in the familiar field with their buddies.

The removal of mares continues until the last foals have been weaned. This method works best with a group of several mares and foals, but you can also use it when there are just two or three mares with foals in a pasture. The first mare to be removed should always be the mother of the most independent foal, the one who has shown all the signs that he is ready to be weaned (see box).

With **stall or barn weaning,** the mare and foal to be weaned are first brought into the barn and fed. After eating and staying inside for a few hours, the foal stays in the stall while the mare is taken to a distant pasture where she can't hear or see her foal. Feed tubs and anything else a foal can run into are taken out of the stall before the mare is removed. It is helpful to play a radio in the barn so the foal can't hear his mother neighing as she is led away. It may help if your vet gives the foal a light tranquilizer before the mare is removed from the stall.

Although it may seem that newly weaned foals won't be so lonely if there are two foals in one stall, studies show this situation actually to be more stressful than being alone. Let each foal have his own stall if you choose this weaning method, a familiar one in which he has been fed with his mother in the past. The weanlings should be able to see and hear each other so they don't feel abandoned.

Most people who use this weaning method keep the foal inside the stall for a week or so before turning him back out. If the foal is turned back outside the same day as weaning, there is a greater chance of him getting injured from racing around trying to find his mother. Keeping the foal inside for several days also allows you to spend extra time handling and working with him.

If you have several foals, once they have quieted down and accepted the separation, you can turn them out in a group. It is best to keep together foals that were in the same pasture before weaning, as they will already be buddies. Fillies and colts can be separated at a later date.

Weaning Issues to Consider

Evaluate the mare and foal's environment before weaning, using the following criteria:

- Is the fencing safe and solid?
- Is the farm large enough that mare and foal can be separated without seeing or hearing each other? If not, where can the mare be boarded temporarily for weaning?
- Are there other foals to be weaned about the same time? If there are no other foals, is there a buddy (a quiet old pony, a trustworthy "babysitter" horse, a burro, or a goat) to keep the new weanling company?
- Are there other horses the mare can be safely put with after weaning?
- Will you or another reliable horse person be able to check on the mare and foal regularly, especially during the first few days after weaning?

Separation Issues

For weaning to go smoothly, mare and foal need to be in separate places where they can't possibly see or hear each other. If you have only one mare and foal and do not have the farm acreage to keep them well apart, try to arrange to board the mare at another farm or stable for a month or so. If you just take her out and put her in a nearby pen or pasture, she and her foal can hear each other's calls and may try to go through or over fences to reunite. Then you may have an injured horse and a vet bill to deal with, in addition to weaning problems.

In the case of the lone foal, the best situation is to have a "babysitter" on hand that the foal is already familiar with when you're ready to let him out of the stall. Talk with your vet before weaning. She may know of someone who has an older pony or reliable horse that is safe with young horses that you can lease or borrow for a few weeks. Weaning is much harder on a foal if he is left alone after his mother is taken away. Horses are herd animals and need companionship.

After you bring back the mare, put her in a separate fenced area, or the newly weaned foal may try to start nursing again. Some mares won't allow, but others will; to be on the safe side, keep them separated, or you will have to go through the weaning process all over again.

Weaning Safety

Many of the same safety precautions you took when preparing the foaling area apply to weaning the mare and foal. Remove anything potentially hazardous from the foal's stall or pen. Fencing should be strong, solid, and safe. Under no circumstances should you use barbed wire, smooth wire, or electric fencing to separate mares and foals at weaning time.

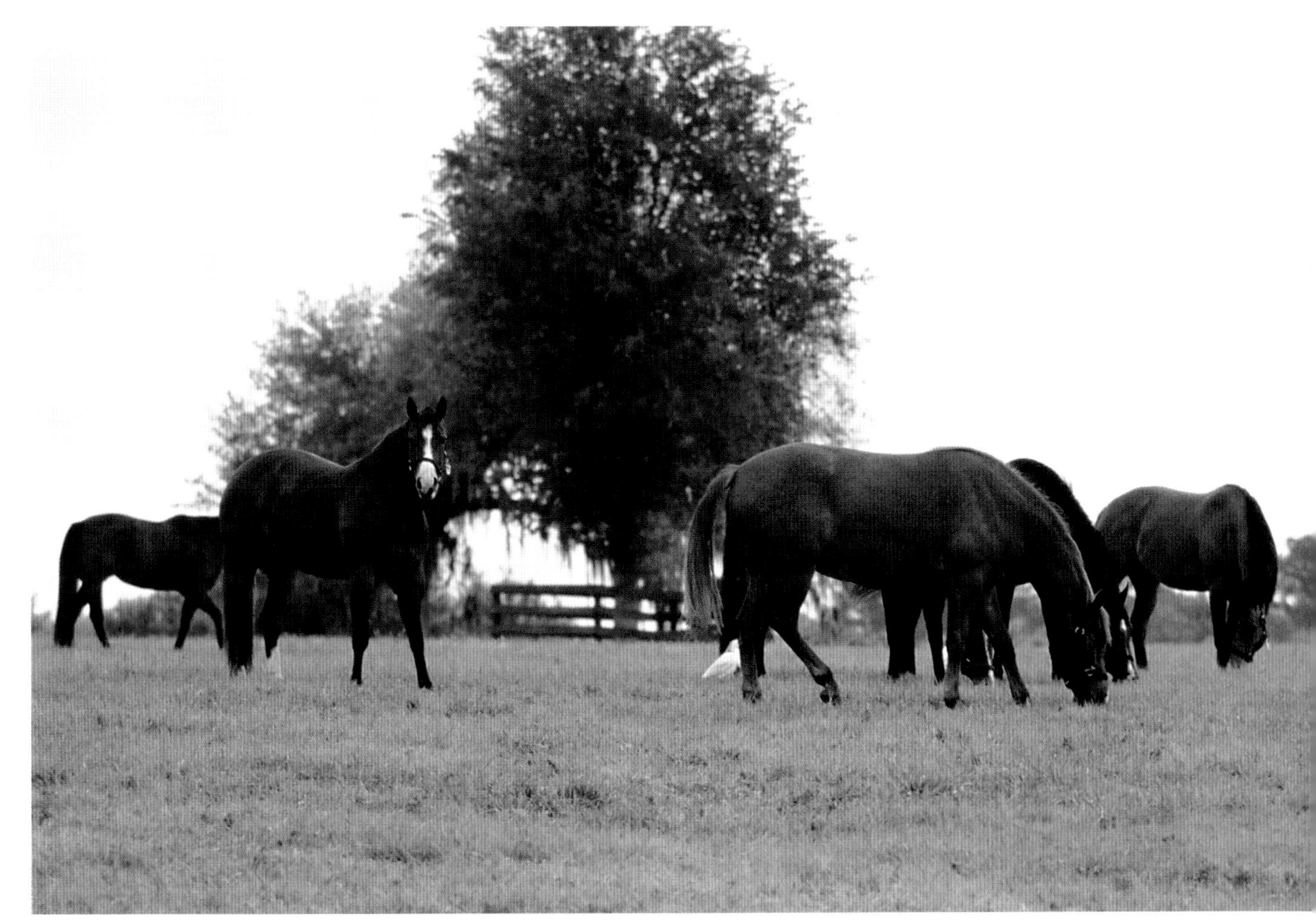

Weaning will be easier on the mare if she can be with other familiar horses.

Remove the foal's halter whenever he is loose in his stall, pen, or pasture. Put on his halter for grooming and handling sessions.

If you are stall weaning, don't stay in the stall or pen with the foal immediately after his mother is taken away. He may race around and kick out, and you can observe him safely and just as well right outside the stall or enclosure.

The First Days of Separation

Keep a close eye on your foal, particularly during the week after weaning, to make sure he is eating and drinking normally. Take his temperature daily. The foal may experience stress, and an elevated temperature is usually the first sign of illness or infection. If this is detected promptly, the vet can monitor and treat him if necessary.

Many foals quickly settle into their new role as a weanling. Others take longer, depending on their personality. Follow your customary feeding routine so your foal doesn't have adjustments to make on top of the separation.

Care of the Mare after Weaning

Because your mare has been a milk-producing machine for the past several months, you must watch her closely after weaning. To make sure that she "dries up" as soon as possible, do not feed her grain for the first few days after weaning. You're not trying to starve her; you just want to reduce the calories enough to cut her milk production.

The mare can eat free-choice hay or pasture during this period. Good forage, a vitamin/mineral supplement, salt, and plenty of fresh water are all she needs immediately after her foal is weaned.

Although the mare will be uncomfortable as her udder fills and the foal is not present to nurse, this discomfort lasts only a few days. The amount of time required to dry up varies: some mares dry up almost immediately; others keep producing milk for some time. You'll have to monitor your mare regularly to see how she is doing.

Check the udder daily to be sure the mare hasn't developed **mastitis,** a painful inflammation of the udder. Signs of mastitis include:

- Fever
- An udder that is hot to the touch
- Swelling (often just on one side)
- A yellowish, oozing substance that is not milk

Have your vet examine the mare if she shows any of these signs. If the mare develops mastitis and it is not treated, she can become very ill and her udder may suffer permanent damage.

Once the mare no longer produces milk, you can feed her grain again. Provide a maintenance-level ration, not the high-protein and large amount of feed she received while lactating. Even if she has been bred back and is pregnant again, a maintenance ration is standard at this stage.

Some mares maintain their weight well after weaning and may not even need any grain. In this case, good quality forage, salt, and a vitamin/mineral supplement should be sufficient.

Do not neglect the mare's vaccination, deworming, and hoof-care programs. If she is pregnant again, be particularly attentive to the vaccines the mare should receive in the first and second trimesters. (See recommendations for vaccinations in chapter 1.)

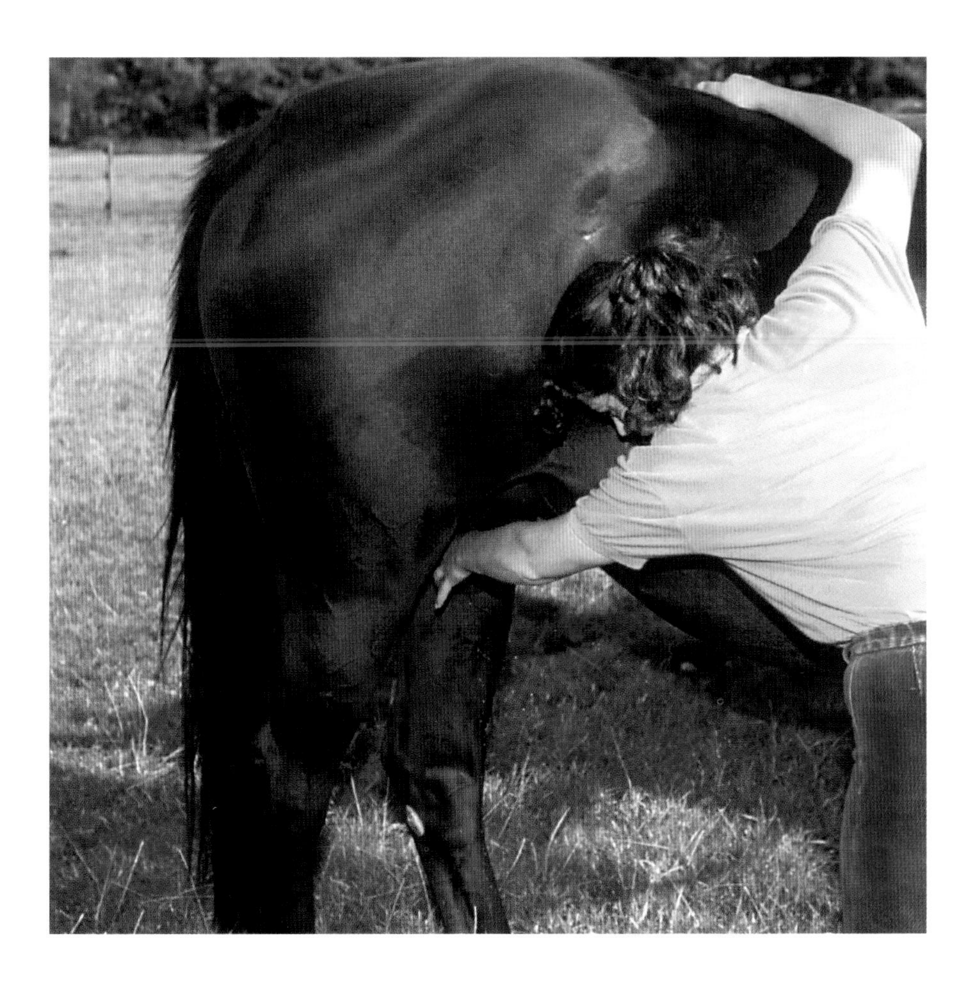

Check the weaned mare's udder daily to make sure mastitis is not a problem.

Nutrition for the Weanling

Foals are typically weaned from midsummer to early fall, depending on their age and readiness. Since birth, a foal's digestive system has developed from processing only milk as the predominant source of nutrition to the more complex demands of forage and concentrate, as the foal grazes and eats hay and grain.

After 3 months of age, the foal still nurses from his dam, but the majority of his nutritional needs are met by the concentrate and forage you provide. A 6-month-old foal will still nurse from his mother if he is not yet weaned, but this activity is more of a comfort behavior than a result of the need to meet any nutritional needs.

By weaning time, the foal should be regularly consuming several pounds of concentrate per day, in addition to forage. Remember, don't feed a foal more than one pound of concentrate per month of age. For example, a 5-month-old foal can be eating up to 5 pounds of concentrate per day, but this is on the upper end of most feeding recommendations. The "1 pound of feed per month of age" suggestion applies only up to age 6 months. You shouldn't be feeding a weanling more than eight pounds of concentrate per day, even if he is 10 months old. *The average weanling should be eating from 1/2 pound to 1 1/4 pounds of concentrate per 100 pounds of body weight per day.*

If you have been feeding a quality concentrate designed for growing foals while the foal is a **suckling,** or nursing foal, continue to follow the feeding recommendations after weaning.

Many commercial concentrates are formulated so that the horse must consume at least 4 pounds of feed in order to receive the entire advertised percentages of nutrients, vitamins, and minerals. If your horse is an easy keeper and you are feeding only 2 pounds of feed daily, you are shortchanging him on his daily requirements. In this case, a vitamin and mineral supplement is called for.

Ration balancers are feeds with a high percentage of protein, and are designed to be fed in small amounts. They are useful when feeding an easy keeper, as they supply the horse's daily nutritional requirements without having to feed a high-volume (of several pounds) concentrate.

Trace mineral salt should be available free choice. Because horses have tongues like those of people, not rough tongues like cows, loose mineral and salt are preferred over blocks. Offer trace mineral salt free choice in a tub or feeder where it cannot get wet. Although commercial feeds contain salt and mineral supplements, horses in humid conditions and those under stress may require even more salt than the average recommended daily amount. If you live in an especially hot and humid climate, ask your vet about adding electrolytes to the feed during the summer to help replace what is lost by sweating.

What about Supplements?

When you visit the feed store and see shelves stocked with supplements, it is tempting to add them to your horse's feed ration. Equine nutritionists, however, caution against randomly feeding supplements. Instead, add them to a horse's feed only when something is missing from the diet or to correct a specific problem. A horse with poor hooves, for example, can

Keep It Balanced!

If you are feeding a balanced commercial ration designed for young horses, be wary of adding oats or other grains. Feed companies formulate and package equine feeds to be used without the need for additional grains or supplements. Oats, for example, are a good source of energy, but they are low in vitamins and minerals and are not balanced in calcium and phosphorus. If you are feeding a balanced commercial feed and add oats to it, you are "unbalancing" the ration. Your best bet is to feed a commercial ration specifically designed for your horse's needs and that the weanling can continue with until he is a yearling.

Horses fare best on a consistent diet. Unlike humans, they don't get bored eating the same ration day after day.

Ideally, your weanling will now be on pasture, where most of his nutritional needs can be met by grazing. If this is not possible or you do not have adequate pasture, provide access to quality hay, fed free choice so he can eat whenever he wants. Alfalfa-mixed grass hay, such as timothy/alfalfa or orchard grass/alfalfa, is usually the best choice. It is not advisable to feed weanlings unlimited straight alfalfa hay because of the high amount of protein and calcium it contains.

benefit from a supplement designed to improve hoof quality.

In some situations, unnecessary supplementation can actually pose a danger to the horse's health. Some vitamins, such as the B vitamins, are water soluble, which means the body can excrete them through urination if they aren't needed. But vitamins A and D are fat soluble and the body will store them. If they are consumed in excess, they can build up to toxic levels. Iron supplements are popular, but the horse's body will absorb iron only when it is needed, and because the body cannot excrete excess iron, it is possible to create dangerously toxic levels in the liver.

If you think your horse needs a supplement, talk it over with the vet before spending money on something your horse may not need or that can cause harm if he consumes too much.

It is important not to make any dramatic revisions in the feeding program at weaning time. Introduce any change in feed gradually over a period of seven to ten days. If the vet suggests a different feeding plan, start changing over the foal to the new routine before or after weaning, but never during.

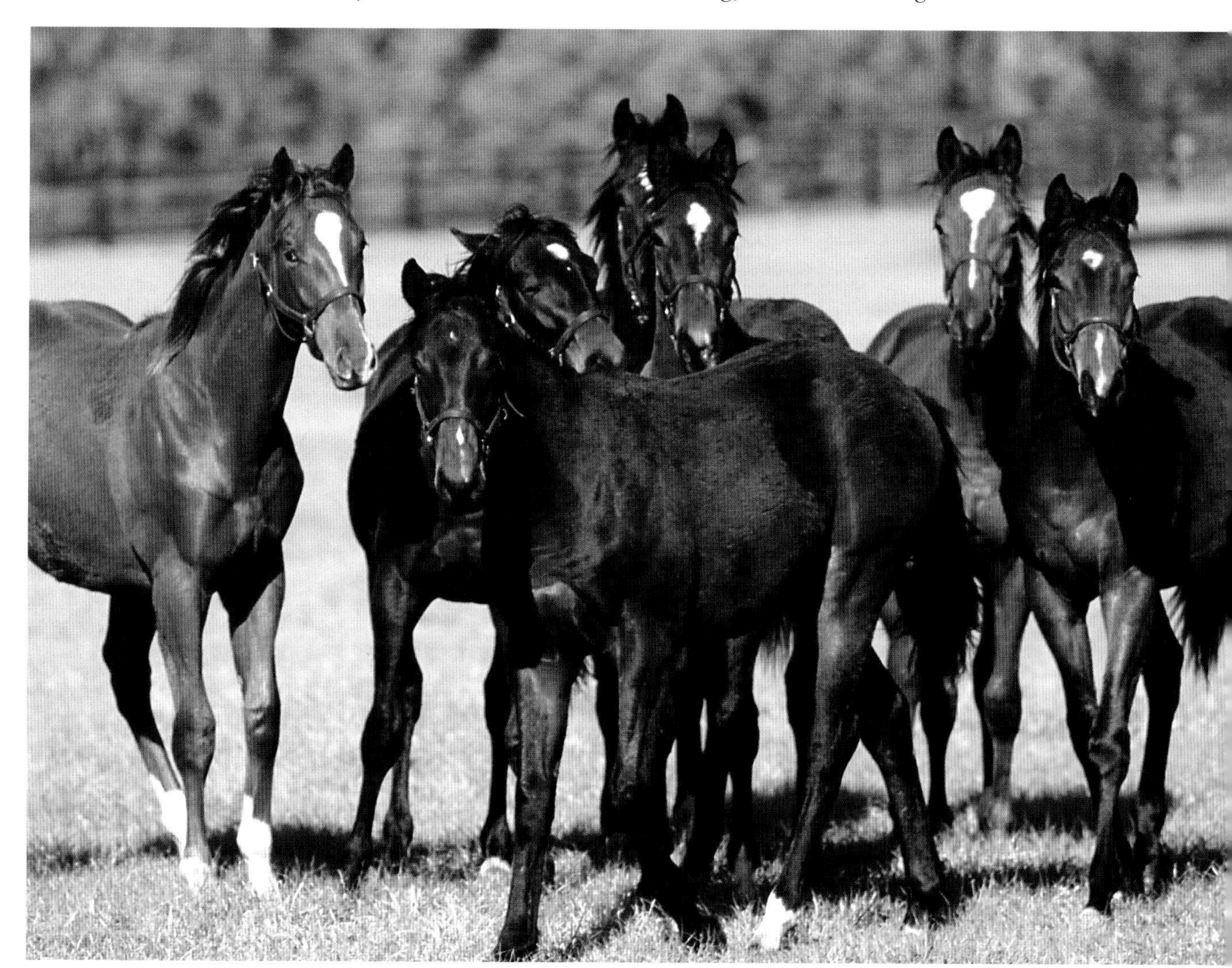

Weanlings should be fed a balanced commercial feed designed for young, growing horses.

10

Growing up Fast

Weanling to Yearling

During the months between weaning and the foal's first birthday, the youngster grows rapidly. In fact, the rate of growth for a horse is highest during his first 12 months of life.

Beyond growing physically, the weanling is maturing mentally and emotionally. This is a prime time to strengthen the partnership you began establishing when he was just a foal. Now that he is no longer pastured with his dam, there are even more activities you can enjoy with the weanling, as his focus will be on you, not his mother. Get ready to expand your horizons and prepare for wonderful adventures as you continue to learn together. While you can't yet ride the young horse at this stage, there are still many things you can do (see page 117) that will increase the bond you have and help prepare him for the day when you *do* step into the saddle.

In the meantime, go on with the regular hoof-care and deworming programs you established when the foal was younger. Add an immunization program to his routine health maintenance if it has not already begun.

Health Care between 6 and 12 Months

During this period you will see numerous changes as your weanling grows rapidly. As you continue to pay close attention to his routine health care and nutrition, you will be giving him the best opportunity to develop properly.

If you have a colt, the period between weaning and his first birthday is usually a good time to have him gelded, if you haven't already had this done. And whether you have a colt or a filly, after weaning is an excellent time to teach him or her to stand tied (see page 112).

Vaccinations

Many of the vaccines recommended for young horses require that the first dose be given at about six months. Some, such as West Nile vaccine, are administered earlier (see chapter 7). Other vaccines, such as influenza, usually aren't given until the foal is about nine months old, due to the vaccinated mare's more powerful and durable antibodies.

The maternal antibodies the foal received through **passive transfer** (drinking his mother's colostrum shortly after birth) can protect him for months. For example, when the mare has been properly vaccinated for equine influenza, the antibodies remain in her foal until he is about 6 months of age. If the foal is vaccinated for influenza while the maternal antibodies are still active, the vaccine will not be effective. The amount of time the antibodies will protect the foal varies, so it is important to discuss with your veterinarian the timing of the foal's vaccination program.

To make sure your foal is adequately protected against infectious equine diseases, the vet will set up a program based on your region and the individual requirements of your horses. The chart on the next page provides a starting point for discussion with your vet about what vaccines your horses need and when. Following up with booster vaccines at the appropriate times is important in order to provide full immunity.

Essential Nutrition

Continue to feed your weanling a quality forage and balanced commercial feed designed for the young, growing horse. Do not switch weanlings and yearlings to adult feed yet, as the nutrients will not be adequate for proper growth and bone development at this stage.

The weanling should be eating 2 to 3 percent of his body weight in feed per day. This amount consists of forage (hay and/or pasture) and concentrate combined. Because the growth rate slows as the horse matures, as a yearling his daily feed intake should only be 1.5 to 2 percent of his body weight.

Always measure feed by weight, not by volume. For example, a flake of loosely compacted grass hay may look larger, but weigh much less, than a small, tightly compacted flake of alfalfa hay does.

Remember to choose your concentrate based on the forage the horse is eating. Some feed rations are designed to complement mainly alfalfa hay–based diets; others are formulated for horses on pasture or eating grass hay. Because alfalfa has much more protein and calcium than grass hay does, the horse eating alfalfa will generally require less protein and calcium in the concentrate. The energy (calories) the horse consumes, not the amount of protein, is what determines his weight gain.

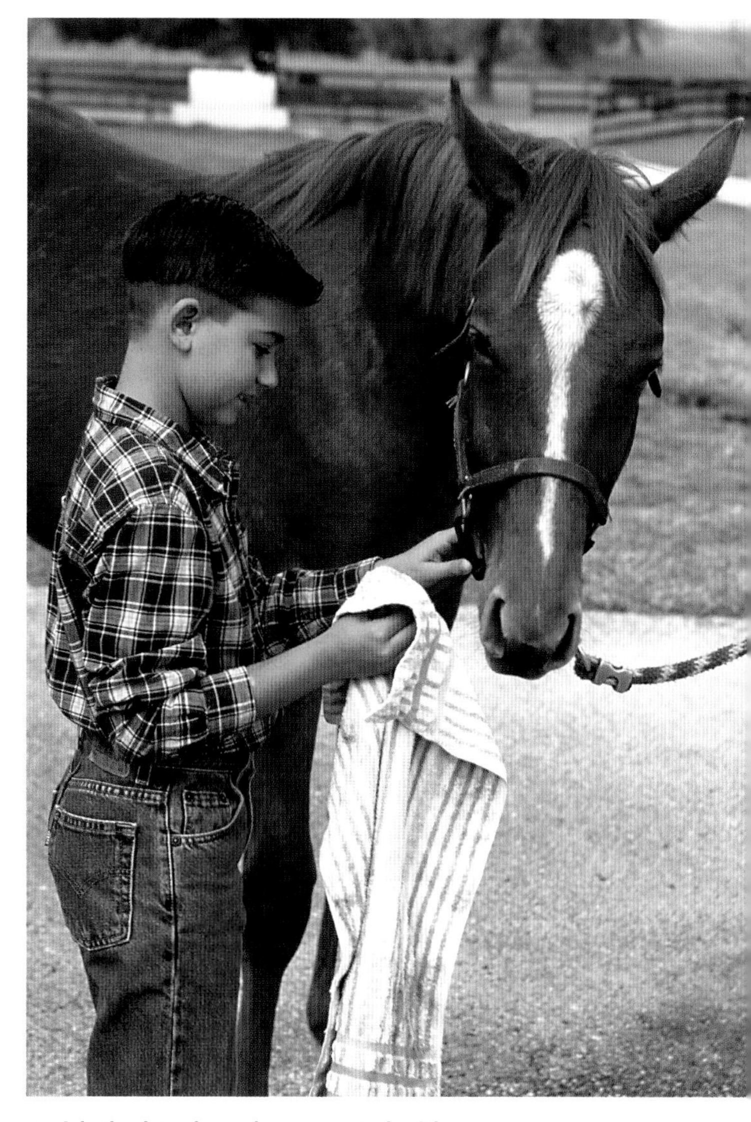

Enrich the bond you have created with your young horse by spending regular time grooming him.

Vaccination Guidelines for Foals and Weanlings

These guidelines, suggested by the American Association of Equine Practitioners (AAEP), are based on standard veterinary practices. Some vaccinations may not be necessary for your particular horse, depending on where you live, the horse's environment, and his medical history.

Recommendations can change, so discuss your specific immunization program with the veterinarian.

Botulism

Vaccinate only where endemic. Timing varies; consult vet.

Equine Encephalomyelitis

Eastern (EEE), Western (WEE),Venezuelan (VEE)

EEE (in high-risk areas):
Give foal first dose at 3–4 months, second at 4–5 months, and third at 5–6 months.

EEE and WEE (in low-risk areas), and VEE:
If mare was vaccinated, give foal first dose at 6 months, second at 7 months, and third at 8 months. If mare was *not* vaccinated, give foal first dose at 3–4 months, second at 4–5 months, third at 5–6 months.

Vaccinate yearlings and older horses annually or twice a year, depending on your area and the vet's recommendations.

Influenza

A series of at least three doses is recommended for primary immunization of foals. Both inactivated injectable and intranasal modified-live-virus vaccines are available.

Inactivated injectable vaccine
If mare was vaccinated, give foal first dose at 9 months, second at 10 months, third at 11–12 months, and then at 3- to 4-month intervals, or as recommended by vet. If mare was *not* vaccinated, give foal first dose at 6 months, second at 7 months, and third at 8 months. Then give at 3- to 4-month intervals, or as recommended by vet.

Intranasal modified live-virus vaccine
Give foal first dose at 11 months. If first dose was given before 11 months, give second dose at or after 11 months of age. Then give at 6-month intervals, or as recommended by veterinarian.

Potomac Horse Fever

Give foals first dose at 5–6 months, second at 6–7 months.

Give semiannually to yearlings and older horses. Where endemic, give booster in May or June.

Rabies

Recommended where endemic. Modified-live-virus rabies vaccines should *not* be given to horses.

Recommendations vary; consult vet. First dose recommended at 3–6 months, followed by boosters. Give annually to yearlings and older horses.

Rhinopneumonitis

Vaccination of mares before breeding and 4–6 weeks prepartum is suggested.

Give foal first dose at 4–6 months, second at 5–7 months, third at 6–8 months. Then give at 3- to 4-months intervals.

Give booster to yearlings and older horses every 3–4 months, up to annually.

Rotavirus A

Little value in vaccinating foals because of insufficient time to develop antibodies during the susceptible age of up to 3 months. To protect the foal, vaccinate broodmares at 8, 9, and 10 months of pregnancy.

Strangles

Administer when risk is high or where it is endemic. Both inactivated injectable and intranasal modified-live-virus vaccines are available.

Injectable vaccine

Give foal first dose at 4–6 months,second at 5–7 months, third at 7–8 months, depending on product used. Fourth dose at 12 months.

Intranasal vaccine

Give foal first dose at 6–9 months, second 3 weeks later. If conditions warrant, foals as young as 6 weeks may receive the intranasal product.

Give semiannually to yearlings and older horses, or as recommended by vet.

Tetanus Toxoid

If mare was vaccinated, give foal first dose at 6 months, second at 7 months, and third at 8–9 months.

If mare was *not* vaccinated, give foal first dose at 3–4 months and second dose at 4–5 months.

Vaccinate yearlings and older horses annually.

West Nile Virus

Recommended in areas where it is endemic.

Give foal first dose at 3–4 months of age, second dose approximately 1 month later, and third dose 6–8 weeks after that.

Give first dose at 3–4 months or younger (as early as 1 month of age), depending on month of birth and mosquito activity. Give second dose approximately 1 month after first, and third dose 6–8 weeks in endemic areas.

Give semiannually to yearlings and older horses, preferably spring and summer/early fall. In areas with an active mosquito population year-round, vaccinate at 3- to 4-month intervals.

A weanling that is expected to mature at about 1,100 pounds should be gaining 1½ to 2 pounds a day at the age of six months. You don't want a weanling to be overly fat or on the thin side (see the body-condition chart on page 3). Use the weight tape to keep track of how much your weanling is gaining, so you can adjust his feed intake accordingly.

As a yearling, the horse will have achieved about 65 percent of his expected weight and almost 90 percent of his expected height. Once the yearling is 12 to 15 months old, both bone and muscle growth rates decline. As a yearling and two-year-old, the horse requires slightly lower levels of protein and minerals, as his growth rate has slowed.

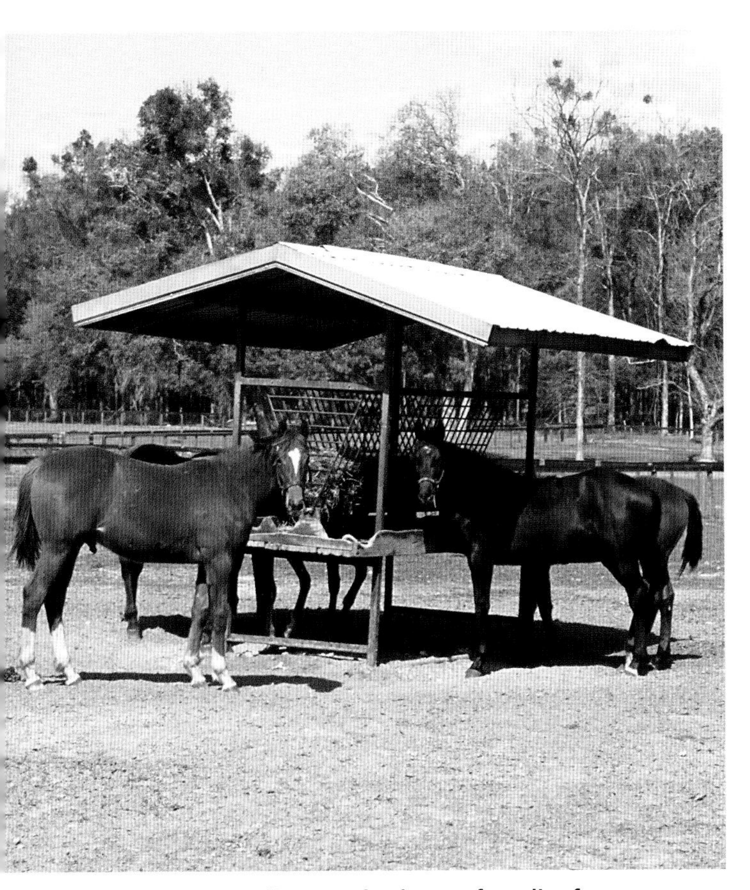

The weanling needs plenty of quality forage.

Separating Colts from Fillies

If you turn out your weanling with other weanlings his age, separate the fillies and colts before there is a chance for them to breed. Most farms separate colts and fillies before they become yearlings. Fillies typically come into their first heat around the age of 1½ years.

Don't wait until the colts start to exhibit "studdish" behavior. Some colts mature earlier than others; a colt may show interest in females as early as 8 or 9 months. There have been numerous cases of yearling fillies becoming pregnant because they were left with the colts, or thanks to a stallion who managed to find his way into the pasture.

If you wean between the ages of 4 and 6 months, let the youngsters recover from any stress of weaning before you separate colts and fillies.

Gelding

Many horse owners don't have the facilities or the experience to keep and handle a stallion. Even the most well-mannered stallion requires attentive handling and strong, secure fencing and stabling.

If you have a colt, now is the time to consider **gelding**, or castrating, him. Geldings usually have an even, reliable temperament and aren't subject to the mood swings and attitudes that stallions and mares can exhibit. Gelding your colt will remove his sexual desire and render him incapable of breeding. It will not limit his development or interfere with his general growth. Contrary to the old wives' tale, it is not necessary to leave a colt intact until he is 2 years old so that he will develop properly. If he receives proper nutrition and health care,

The Gelding Procedure

Although it is possible to geld a colt while he is standing, it is much easier to perform the surgery when the horse is on the ground. Your vet will give the colt an intravenous injection to heavily sedate him before administering an anesthetic. As the anesthetic takes effect, the vet or her assistant holds on to the horse's halter or lead rope to steady him and ease him down to the ground. It will take only a few minutes for the colt to lose consciousness.

With the colt lying flat on his side, the veterinarian disinfects the area and makes an incision in the scrotum to expose the testicles (1). She then crushes the cords to the testicles using a set of **emasculators,** a handheld tool that helps prevent hemorrhage (2). After the initial cut, the site should not bleed much, and when the testicles are removed (3, 4), sutures are not necessary to close up the scrotal sac.

Once the anesthetic wears off, the colt will become conscious of his surroundings and regain his feet, usually within a half hour. Stand clear until he has control of his body and is steady on his feet.

After the first or second day, the vet may tell you to hose the scrotal area gently with a low flow of cold water to reduce swelling and discomfort, and to keep the incision clean and draining. She will advise you when and how often to hose the area. Expect to see some degree of swelling and drainage, but not much if you are carefully following the vet's aftercare instructions. It is also beneficial to turn out the colt so he can move around freely.

Castration is a common procedure with a short recovery and healing period. The incision should be healed within three weeks. Medication is usually not necessary unless there are complications.

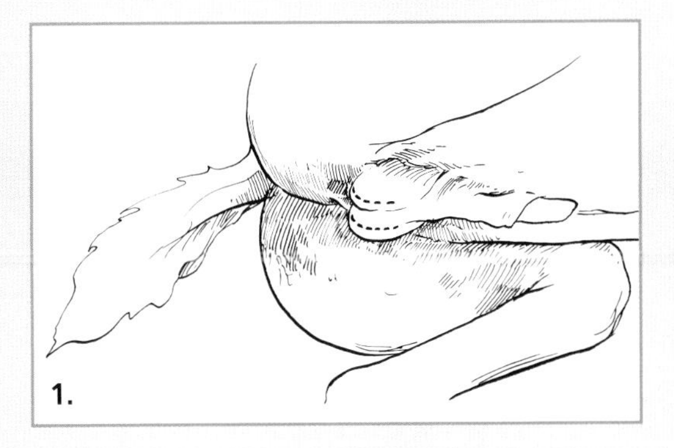

1.

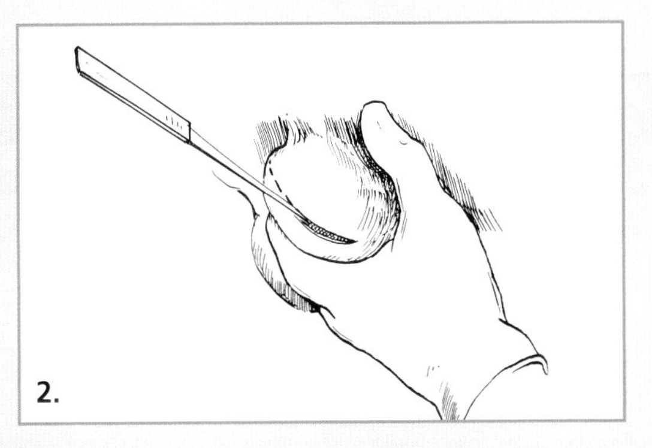

2.

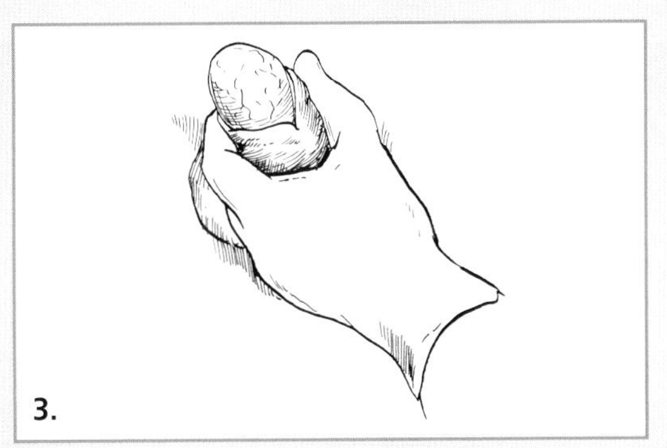

3.

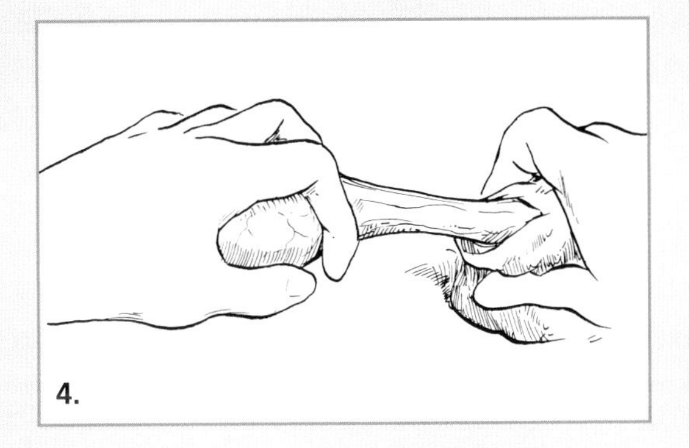

4.

When to Geld

- If both testicles are descended, colt can be gelded younger than 6 months.
- If both testicles have not descended earlier, it is common to geld between the ages of 6 months and 1 year.
- Don't geld during hot weather — spring and fall are better.
- Don't geld if the colt has recently been ill or was just weaned. He should be healthy and not under any stress.

gelding him — even earlier than 6 months — will have no adverse impact on his development.

Many horsemen believe it is easier on the colt to geld him before he even starts thinking about breeding activities. Some owners like to geld before weaning a colt. If the colt is young, gelding is only a minor surgical procedure with a rapid recovery time. If this is your choice, be sure to schedule castration early enough that the animal will have recovered completely before the stress of weaning.

It is also common to geld between the ages of 6 and 12 months. The testicles should have descended (typically, shortly after the colt is born) and be of adequate size by now. With some colts just a few weeks old, it is not unusual for the testicles to draw back up against the abdominal wall and not descend again until the colt is about 1 year old.

In addition to the colt's age and sexual development, the time of year is an important factor. Most veterinarians discourage gelding in very hot weather, as flies present an infection problem. For that reason, spring or fall is the usual recommendation for gelding.

Learning to Tie

Once you have weaned the foal and he is about 6 months old, it's time to teach him to tie. All horses should know how to stand quietly when tied. This is one of the most important lessons a young horse must learn.

Restricting the horse's movement by tying him takes away his most important survival behavior: the ability to flee danger. Panic can ensue if a horse hasn't been taught to tie. He can injure himself if he becomes frightened and pulls back, breaking the halter or rope. It is imperative that you teach him properly: horses have been seriously hurt, and even killed, by being tied to something unstable or on a rope that is too long. When you teach your young horse to tie properly, you may avoid disaster and can be confident that you will be able to tie him safely whenever you need to.

Cryptorchid

A colt is known as a **cryptorchid** if one or both testicles have not descended. With most cryptorchids, only one testicle is evident; the other may be located in the abdominal area. In this case, abdominal surgery is required to remove it. If the testicle remains undescended, the colt will develop and act like a stallion, and he will be able to breed mares even though the testicle is not visible in the scrotum.

Before lessons can begin, your young horse must know how to lead well (see chapter 7). If you have been working with him routinely while he was a suckling, he should be ready to learn to tie after he has been weaned, at about 6 months.

To reinforce your ground work, spend a few sessions in the stall to make sure the weanling is responding to your commands. *Note:* You can begin this lesson before he is weaned, but it is much easier without his mother in the stall. Halter him and hold a longe whip in your right hand and the lead rope in your left. Use voice commands and body language to drive the weanling in a circle around you. If he needs encouragement, move the longe whip behind him or tap the ground just behind his hind legs. *Do not hit or touch the weanling with the whip.*

Conduct this "driving-around-the-stall" lesson in both directions for several days, until you are confident he is responding well.

If you have been consistent with lessons about pressure and release during the previous months, the weanling should learn to tie easily. For example, when you asked the foal to back up by pressing your fingers into his chest, you kept the pressure firm until he backed away. At that point, you immediately released any

Tying the Weaning

Use a strong rope halter with the lead rope braided into it. This combination is recommended because the hardware and snaps on lead ropes and regular halters can break under stress. If you do use a nylon halter, it *must* have heavy-duty hardware, and the lead rope must have an extra-strong snap, such as a brass bull snap.

If the horse pulls back and breaks the halter or lead rope in this first lesson, he will learn that pulling back leads to release of pressure. This is *not* the lesson you want him to learn. If a horse realizes he can pull back and get free once, you can be sure he will try it again. What he must learn is that if he pulls back, the pressure increases and is released only when he steps forward.

It is helpful to have someone on hand when you tie for the first time. That person, standing behind the weanling and off to the side, holds the longe whip.

1. Using the quick-release knot (see page 116), tie the weanling to a solid post, tree, or secure stall tie ring. Always tie short and at least as high as the horse's withers — preferably at or above the horse's head level.

2. Groom or rub the weanling for a few minutes while he is tied. Don't leave him alone. If he starts to pull back, the person with the longe whip flicks it at the ground immediately behind the horse until he steps forward, or gently touches the horse on the hind legs with the whip.

3. A 5- to 10-minute session is enough for the first lesson. Continue to tie him on a regular basis, gradually increasing the time that he stands quietly.

Always keep an eye on the young horse when he is tied. Once the time comes for under-saddle training, when he is older, the horse will already be a pro about tying.

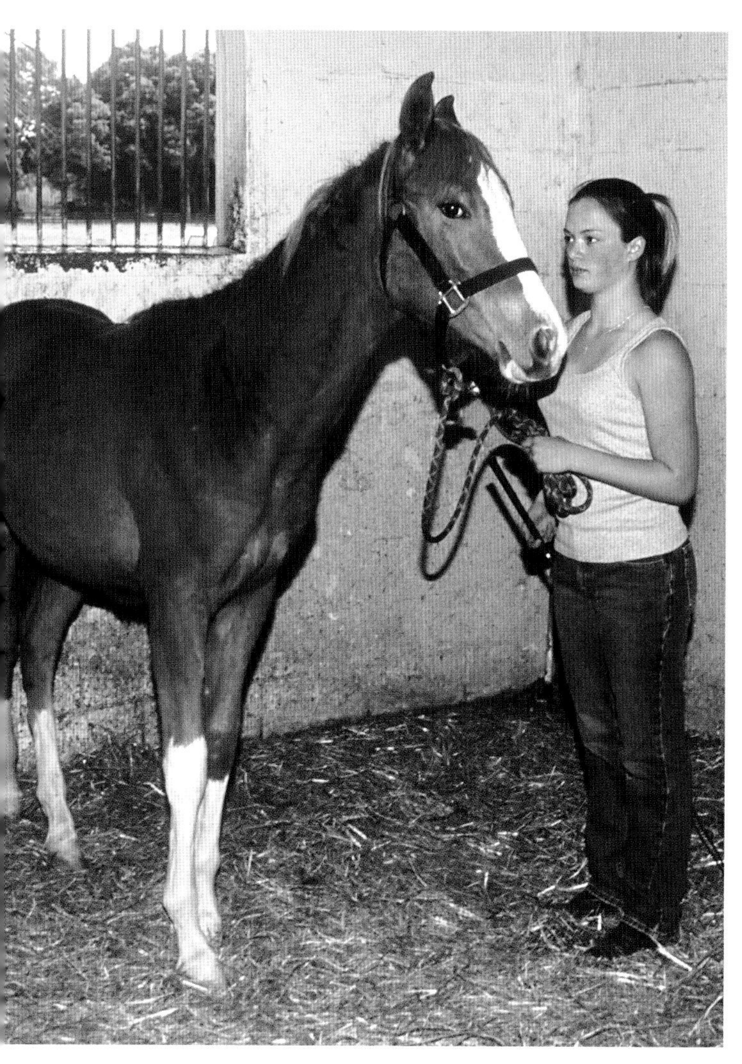

Ground-work lessons in the stall will help prepare your weanling for tying. He should move forward, backward, and sideways at your command.

pressure. The same lesson applies to learning to move forward with the butt rope providing pressure on the hindquarters. By now he should be familiar with the concept that when he responds correctly, pressure is relieved.

Body Rope

If you have consistently followed the handling recommendations in previous chapters, teaching your weanling to tie won't be stressful for either horse or human. There may come a time, however, when you have to work with a horse that hasn't had the thorough preparation you have given your foal from birth. In such a case, it is helpful to use a body rope for the first tying lessons.

Use a body rope only on an older horse to teach him not to pull back when tied.

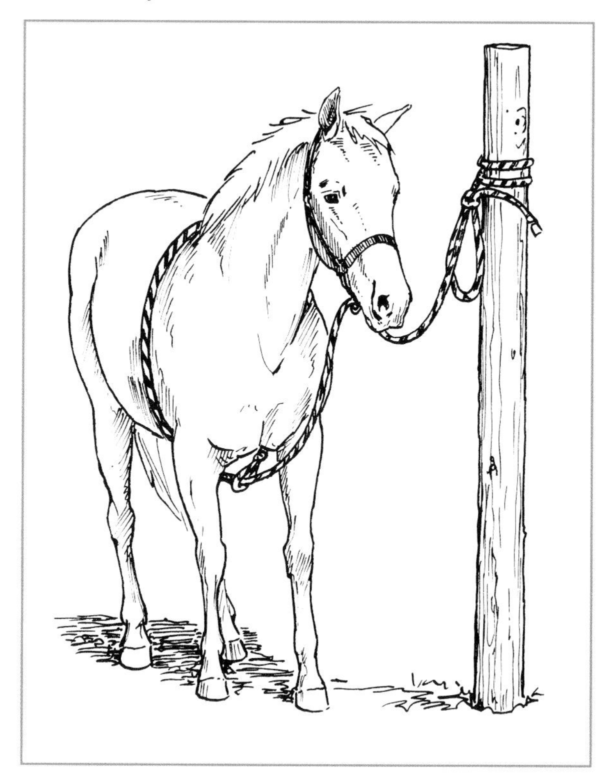

To avoid rubbing, use a thick cotton rope at least 1 inch in diameter. Tie a small loop in one end and put the rope over his back, just behind the withers and around his belly. The loose end of the rope goes through the loop and up between the horse's front legs. In essence, you have made a large slipknot around the horse's body. This is actually a variation on the butt rope, but the rope is placed around the horse's barrel instead.

Bring the loose end between the front legs and through the bottom ring on the halter. If the rope is too thick to pass through the ring, simply run it through the halter's chin strap. Tie the rope short and high to a solid post, tree, or tie ring using the quick-release knot.

With this method, if the horse pulls back, the rope immediately squeezes him around the middle, encouraging him to step forward. As soon as he does so, the pressure is released. Even challenging and fractious horses quickly learn that there is no sense in pulling back.

Once the horse no longer tests the body rope, you can begin tying with a lead rope attached to the halter as usual.

Caution: If and when you do use a body rope, be prepared for the horse to react much more quickly and intensely. Only an experienced horse person should use this method. A body rope should not be used on young foals or weanlings.

Dos and Don'ts of Tying

- *Do* teach the horse to tie in an area with good, secure footing, never on pavement or any surface that may be slippery.
- *Don't* leave tied a horse of any age until you are confident he has learned not to pull back.
- *Do* use a sturdy rope halter or unbreakable nylon halter with heavy-duty hardware; *don't* use a leather halter when teaching to tie, as it may break. A rope halter with the lead rope braided into it is best.
- *Do* tie only to something solid, such as a stout tree or heavy post.
- *Don't* tie to a fence board, rail, wire fence, gate, vehicle, or small tree limb, or anything else that might break or come loose.
- *Do* make sure the immediate area is free of hazards, such as vehicles, stable equipment, and buckets.
- *Do* tie high (head level or higher) and short.
- *Don't* tie so low that the horse's head can reach the ground.
- *Do* use a quick-release knot so you can get the horse untied in an emergency.
- *Don't* tie with a bridle or reins, as this can damage the horse's mouth.

Quick-Release Knot

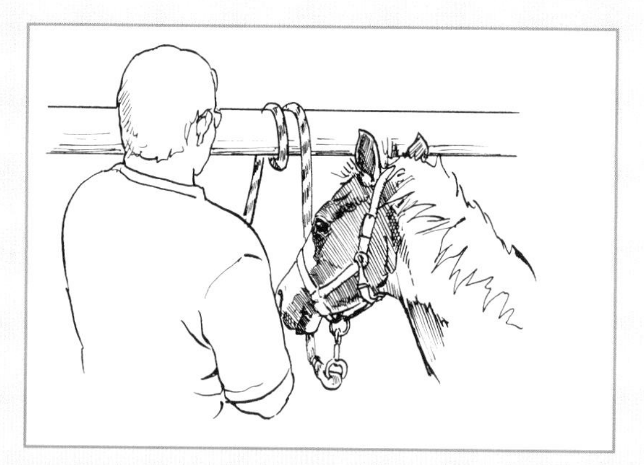

1. Wrap the lead rope two or three times around the ring or post you are tying to. This will prevent the knot from becoming too tight.

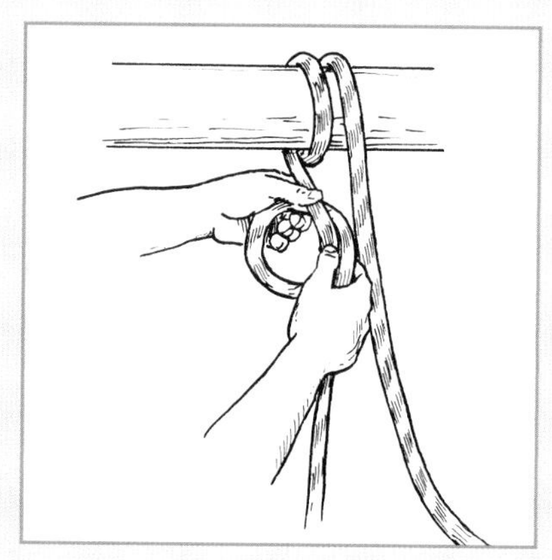

2. Make a small loop in the loose end of the rope.

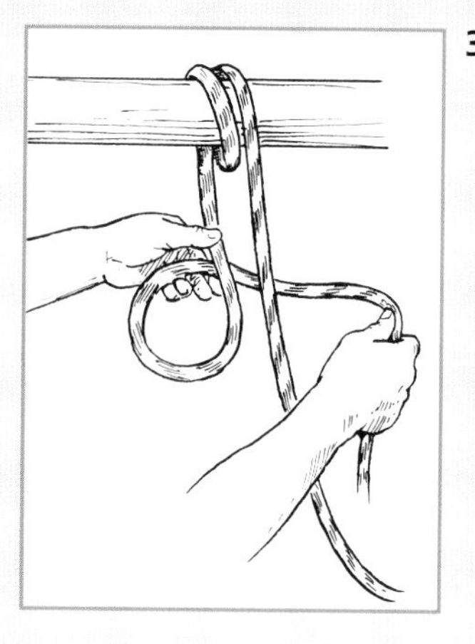

3. Pass the loose end around the attached lead rope, double it, and put the doubled end through the loop.

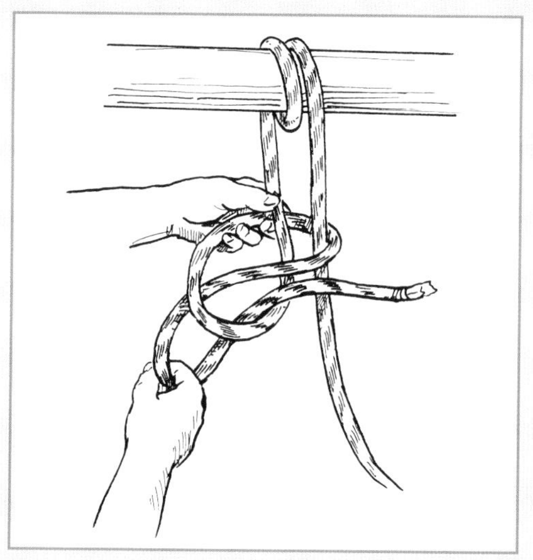

4. Pull the knot snug. (To remember how to make the knot, think, "The rabbit comes out of the hole, goes around the tree, then goes back down the hole again.").

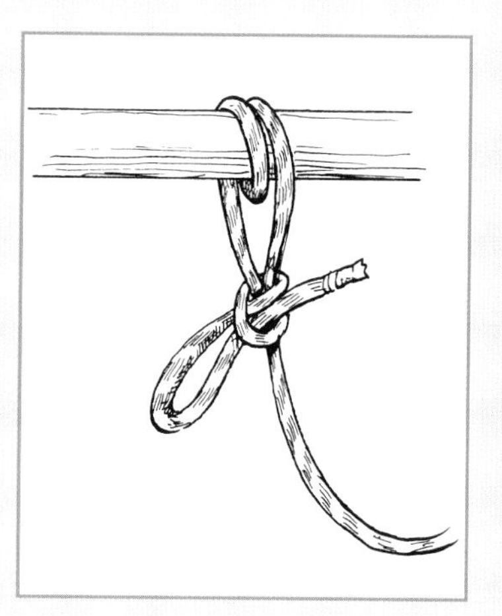

5. You can pull the loose end if you need to release the horse quickly, but he cannot pull the knot loose.

Build Confidence with an Obstacle Course

Once the weanling is accustomed to life without Mom, you are free to do more things with him. Regular handling, grooming, leading, and tying will make him easy to work with. One excellent way to expose the young horse to new things and to build confidence not only in himself but also in you as his handler is to create an obstacle course.

Some shows offer in-hand trail classes in which yearlings compete over an obstacle course similar to those used in under-saddle trail classes. Even if you have no intention of showing in such a class, an obstacle course is a good schooling tool.

A large area is not necessary, nor is expensive or fancy equipment. Everything you need can be purchased at a home supply or hardware store.

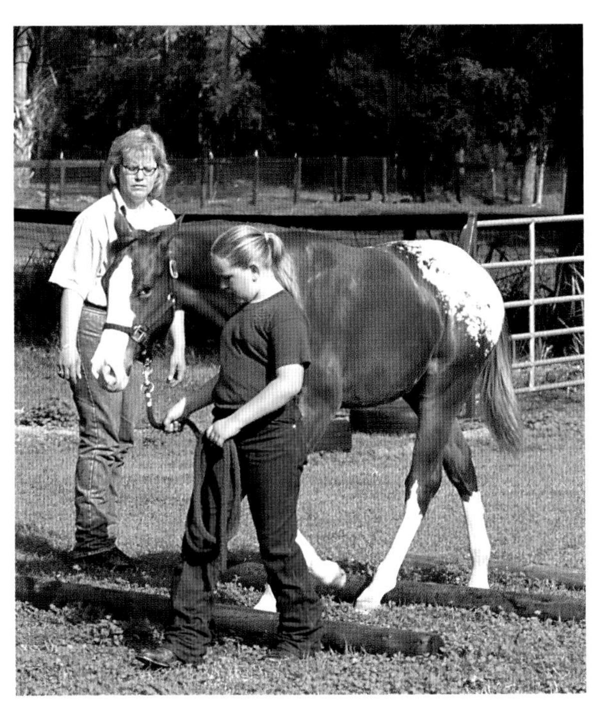

Build the young horse's confidence with an obstacle course.

Here's what you need to make your own obstacle course:

- Landscaping posts, rails, or cavalletti poles
- Plastic orange highway safety cones (they don't have to be large)
- Pressure-treated 2 × 6 or 2 × 8 lumber (for bridge)

Focus on what's Working!

As you are bound to discover if you haven't already, horse ownership can be humbling. These magnificent animals can evoke a range of emotions in their human caretakers, ranging from elation and satisfaction to anger and frustration.

Always remember, the horse isn't trying to upset you or make you mad. When our horses don't respond the way we desire, it is because they either don't understand what we are asking, or they are looking for an easier way to do it.

The horse will happily let you be his leader if he feels he can trust you. However, he will still look for the easiest way to do whatever it is you ask. This is why you must make your requests clear and always build on what the horse knows.

Remember, whatever you focus on is what you will get more of! If you continue to "drill" on what is making him anxious, he will simply become more anxious. Back up to something he is confident about and *gradually* introduce new and different things, step by step.

Lay Out the Course

Design a simple course so that your weanling must walk over several poles on the ground, weave through four plastic cones, and walk over a bridge. It's okay to concentrate all the obstacles in a fairly small area. Because the goal is to introduce the weanling to new experiences, building his confidence as you go, the obstacle course should be a fun lesson, never a power struggle.

Ground Poles

The first step is to introduce him to poles on the ground. Standing at his left shoulder, where you would typically lead him, walk the weanling up to a pole on the ground. Allow him to lower his head and sniff the pole as much as he wants. Then use a clucking sound to encourage him to move forward, and walk him over the pole.

The first few times, he may try to sidepass and avoid the pole, but he will soon realize that it is nothing to worry about. Praise and rub him when he walks over it.

Cones

Set up four plastic cones in a straight line, with several feet between each cone. Walk the weanling through them in a weaving pattern.

Walking over poles on the ground will help your weanling pay attention and learn that he can tackle new things.

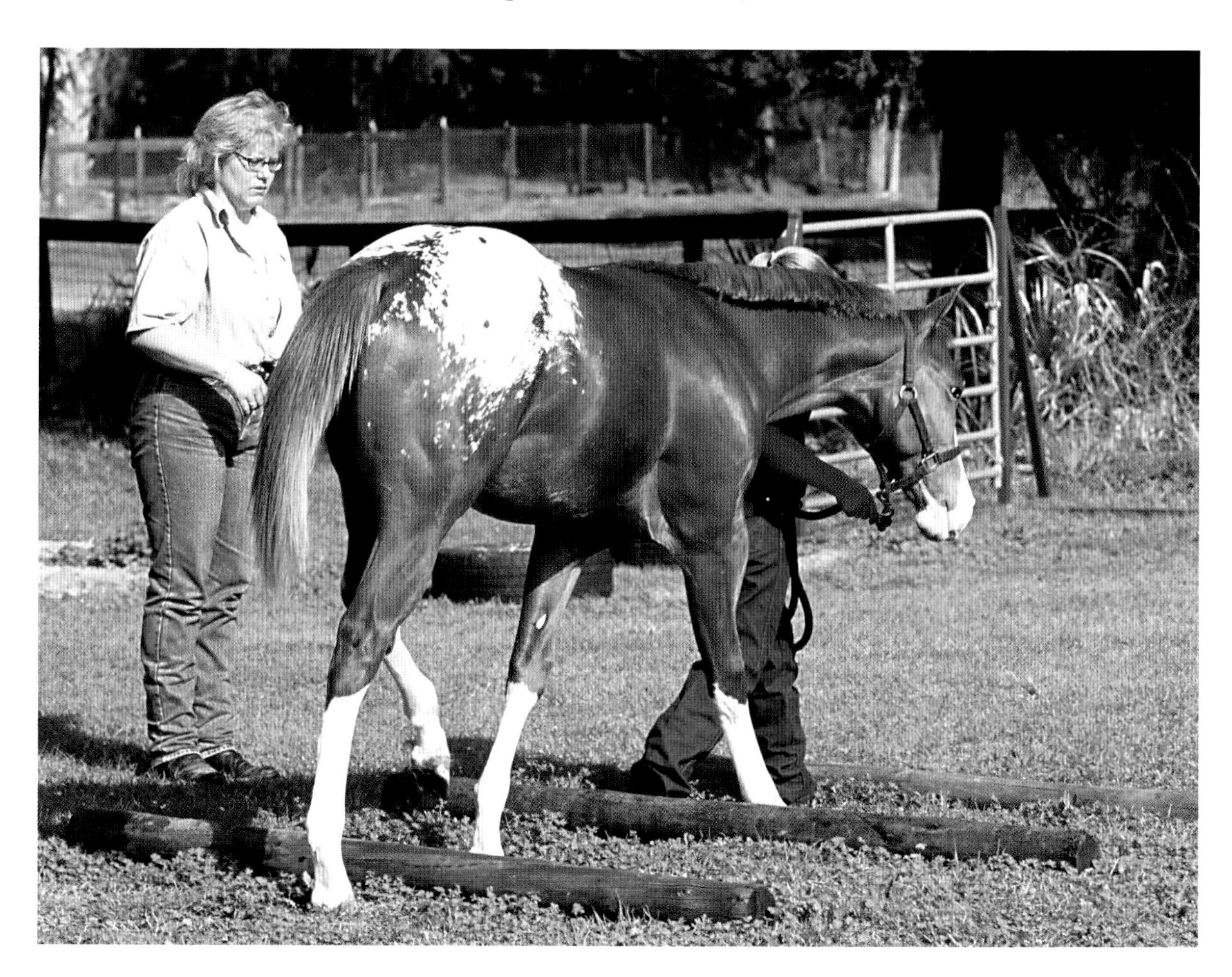

Always approach an obstacle head-on, so that the weanling is facing it and his body is straight. This will give him a greater chance of success.

Bridge

Take your time when asking the weanling to walk over an obstacle such as a bridge, and don't introduce this until he has mastered walking over several poles in a row. Remember how your horse experiences new things. Allow him to drop his head and sniff the lumber, and don't become impatient.

The sound of his hooves on the wood may startle the weanling when he first steps onto the bridge. If he steps off the side, calmly walk him around to face the bridge head-on again. If the weanling learned to load into a trailer with a ramp when he was a foal, he should catch on to navigating the bridge without difficulty.

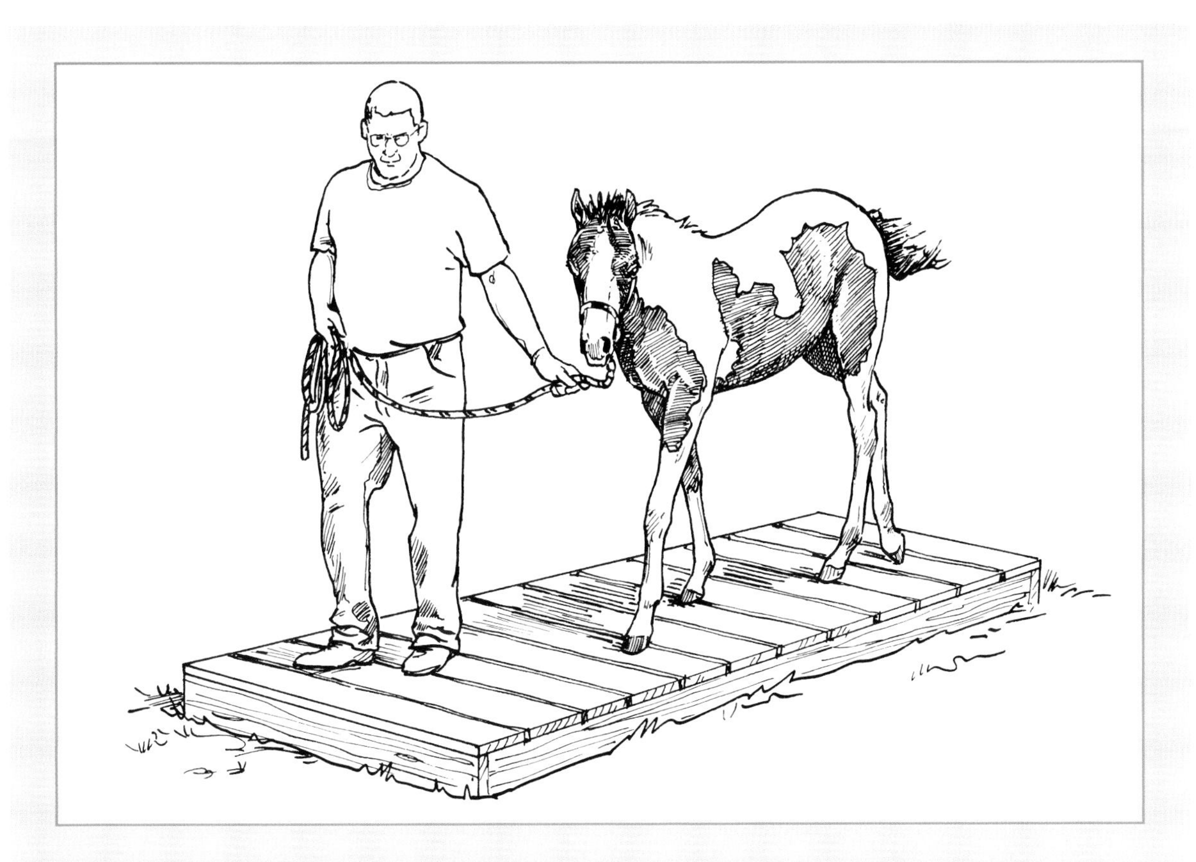

Build a Bridge

Walking over a small bridge is a good learning experience for the weanling. He must learn to step up onto a strange object and walk across it. Make sure the bridge is strong and sturdy, so the horse feels confident when putting his weight on it.

The bridge should be 4 to 5 feet long and no less than 3 feet wide. Use pressure-treated 2 × 6 or 2 × 8 pine or oak boards. First build a framework of boards, then nail or screw down the top boards horizontally, leaving about ½ inch of space between boards. Sink all nail or screw heads into the boards so that all wood surfaces are smooth.

Rewards and Next Steps

When the weanling masters an obstacle, praise him by rubbing him and speaking in soothing tones. If you are going to give him any treats, such as bites of carrot, save this until you are finished; otherwise, the weanling may become pushy and focus more on snacks than on what you are asking him to do.

Once the weanling has mastered each obstacle, you can add variety by changing the sequence or asking him to try other exercises. Position barrels or more cones to weave among, and try backing him up between two poles on the ground. Add a large inflatable ball to the obstacle course, or use a garden hose to design a weaving "trail" to walk through. Spread a plastic tarp flat on the ground and teach the horse to walk over it. As long as the obstacles don't present a danger to you or the horse, you can introduce a variety of things to the course. Learning to negotiate these different obstacles will develop your horse's confidence and make it easier for him to accept new things.

Keep it safe and remember to think like a horse when introducing an obstacle. Don't make this a daily drill. After the weanling is comfortable with the course, just take him through it once or twice a week. Vary the sequence of the obstacles so the course doesn't become predictable or boring.

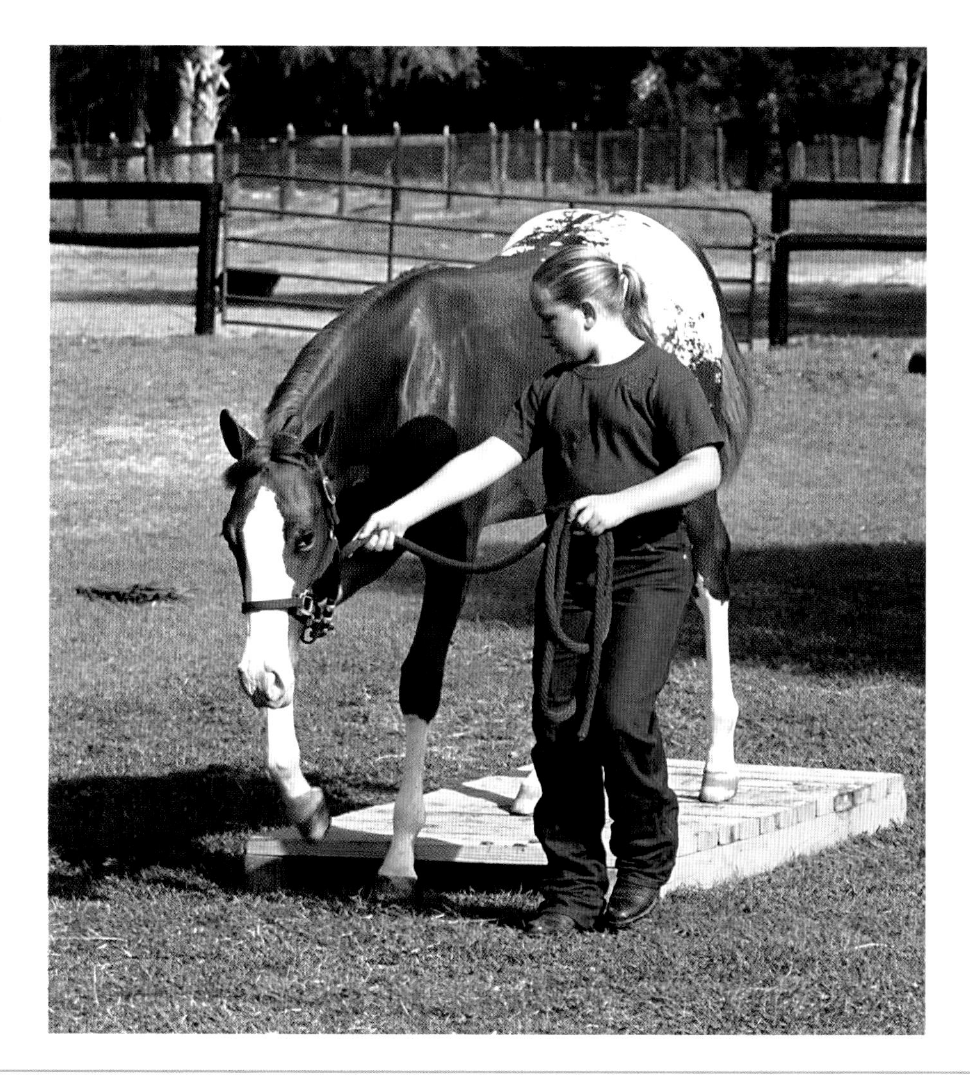

Approach obstacles head-on and be patient. Give the weanling time to master each obstacle, and praise him when he succeeds.

11

Paperwork Time:

Naming and Registration

If you have a purebred foal, registration is usually done within the first year. Most registries charge a fee that is less expensive the younger the horse is, so be sure to check with your breed registry.

Naming Your Foal

Chances are your foal is already named. If you haven't yet decided on a formal name, you have no doubt come up with at least a barn name or nickname that the foal recognizes. Although your horse won't care if his name is Glue Stick or something much more dignified, you will.

Many owners believe in giving their horses names they can "live up to." If you plan to enter competitions with him, consider how the name will sound over the public address system at a show or meet. Some owners go for cute and catchy; others want something grand and memorable.

When registering your foal, you will need to come up with his official name at the time you fill out the paperwork. This can be more difficult than it sounds, as even some unusual names have been taken and are therefore ineligible for your foal.

Rules vary among registries. At publication time, the American Quarter Horse Association (AQHA), the world's largest equine breed registry, with more than four million horses registered, allows up to 20 characters in a name, including spaces. Punctuation marks are not allowed, nor are sound-alike versions of names already in use. Most registries won't accept inappropriate or suggestive names either.

Trademarked names and copyrighted names, such as song titles, aren't allowed without written permission from the copyright holder. If you want to name your foal after a famous person, you must get his or her written permission.

Some registries will allow a name to be used only once, even if the original horse died long ago. Other registries will let a name be used again, provided it was not a famous horse. In other words, there will never be another Thoroughbred named Secretariat!

Most breed registries allow you to submit a number of choices. Always list names in order of your preference: the first available name is the one your foal will receive. Many owners like to use some combination of the sire's and dam's names, but you can come up with a completely original name for your foal.

If you are at a loss as to what to name your foal, feel free to call the registry; someone on staff will be able to help you.

Colors and Markings

When you are filling out the registration paperwork, carefully note the foal's markings, if any, and his color. Recognized colors vary depending on the breed and registry. For example, The Jockey Club, which registers Thoroughbreds, does not recognize sorrel but does list chestnut.

Defining your horse's color isn't always simple, as coloration may be tricky to determine. The difference between gray and roan, for example, can be confusing. Gray horses will change color as they age and are typically born very dark or almost black. Both gray and roan horses have dark skin, but on a roan foal, the ears are always a solid color. With a gray foal, white hair will increase on the face as the foal ages, especially around the eyes and on the ears. One or both parents must be gray in order for the foal to be considered gray. The same is true with roan and dun coloring.

Misunderstandings about colors are common. If you are uncertain as to your foal's exact color, contact the registry. Many people think they have a black horse when the horse is actually brown or dark bay. A true black horse is black all over, including the muzzle and flanks, may not have white markings. Some sorrel horses have a dorsal stripe, but that doesn't make them duns.

Some breeds, such as the Appaloosa and the American Paint Horse, are known for their

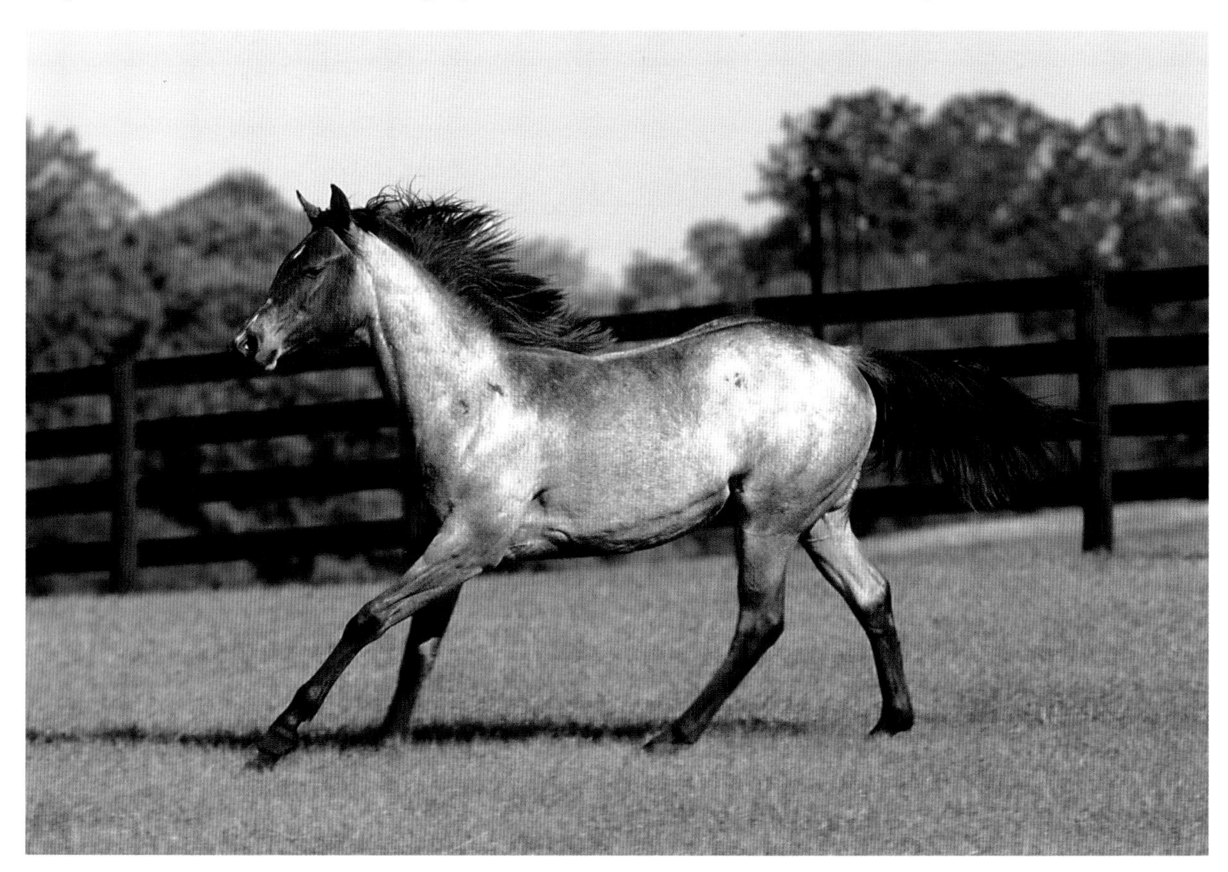

A roan, as shown here, will always have solid-colored ears; a gray foal will usually have white hair on the face, especially around the ears and eyes.

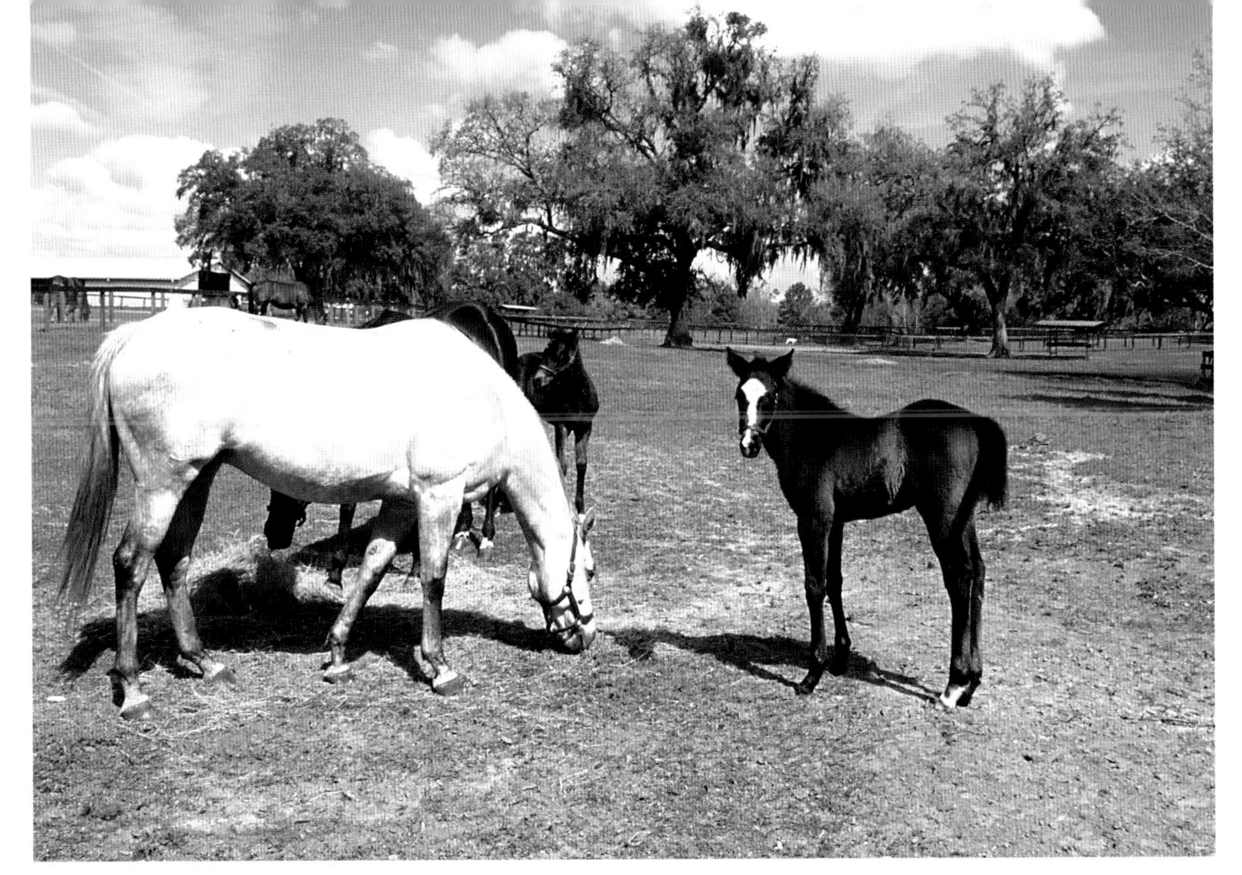

This nearly black filly will mature to be a gray, like her dam.

colorful coat patterns. Their breed registries recognize specific colorations, patterns, and markings, and in both breeds a horse is sometimes born solid-colored.

Appaloosa patterns combine white with another solid color. Spots vary in size from small specks to 3 or 4 inches in diameter. Spots may be found over the entire body (leopard pattern), over the body and hips, over the back and hips, over the loin and hips, or just over the hips. Appaloosas typically have a white sclera, the part of the eye that encircles the iris, and their skin is mottled. Their hooves have boldly defined light and dark vertical stripes.

American Paint Horses usually have one of three recognized coat patterns. In the **tobiano,** the dark color often covers one or both flanks; legs are usually white below the knees and hocks. In the **overo,** white usually doesn't cross the horse's back; at least one and often all legs are dark. In the **tovero,** one or both eyes are blue. There is usually dark pigmentation around the ears and mouth; spots may occur on chest, flanks, barrel and loins.

Photos may be requested for registration to show color and markings. Depending on the particular registry's requirements, you may need to take photos of the horse from both sides, the front, and the back.

A foal's coat color can look different once he sheds his "baby" hair. Refer to the illustrations that follow, and if you still have questions about your foal's exact color, contact the breed registry or some of the Web sites or books listed in the appendix. Depending on your breed, not all of the colors shown may be recognized.

Common Horse Colors

Shown here are many, but not all, of the commonly recognized horse colors. Keep in mind that even within one color category, there are often wide variations. For example, Roy Rogers's Trigger was a rich golden palomino, and people often mistakenly assume that all palominos are this same shade, but there are many horses with a pale "buttery" coloring that definitely qualify as palomino.

Interestingly, not all breed registries recognize the same colors. For example, you could have a Thoroughbred that is registered as a chestnut, while his exact color could qualify as sorrel if he were a Quarter Horse.

Your specific breed registry can answer questions about colors, and there are a number of helpful books and Web sites on horse colors. (See appendix.) And if you happen to have a **grade,** or unregistered, horse, it's up to you to define exactly what color he is!

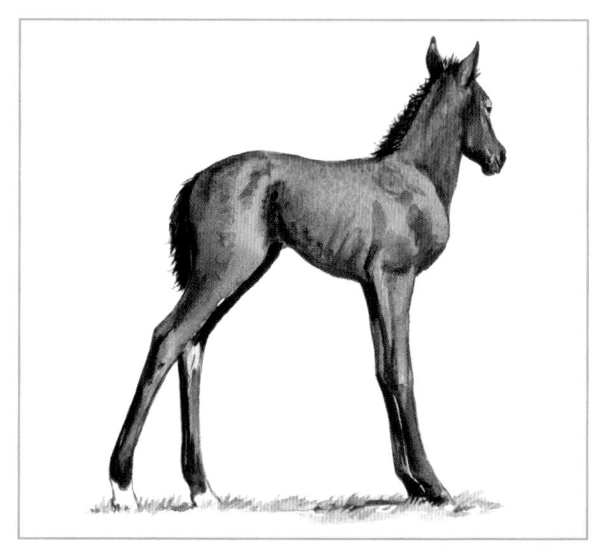

Bay. Ranges from light tan to bright reddish brown. Horses with a rich mahogany shade are known as dark bay. Mane and tail are black, and there is black on lower legs.

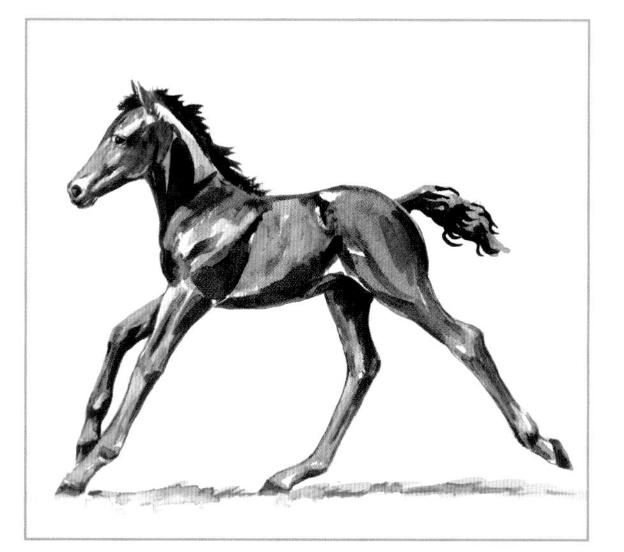

Black. Body, mane, and tail are true black without any light brown areas (excluding white markings).

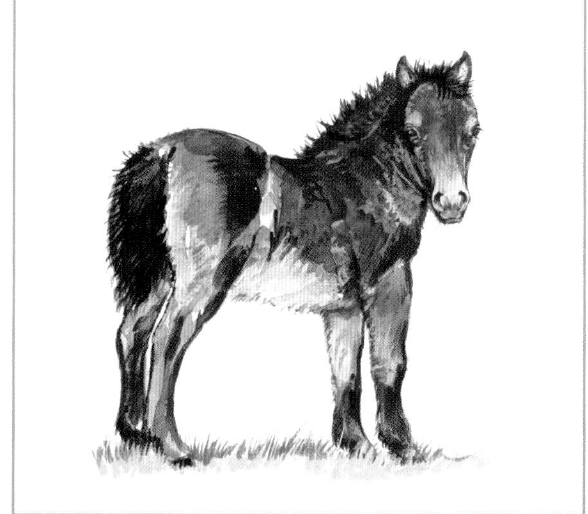

Brown. Color of body ranges from rich brown to almost black, with light areas around the eyes, muzzle, and flanks. Mane and tail are black.

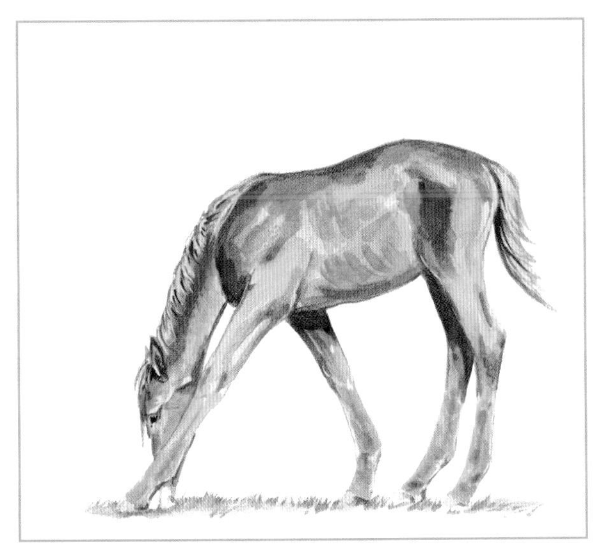

Chestnut. Ranges from orange-red or yellowish red to a deep liver color, with mane and tail usually the same, although they may be flaxen. Even if mane and tail are blackish, the lower legs will be red. (Depending on the breed registry, chestnut may be similar to sorrel, but there is no dorsal stripe.)

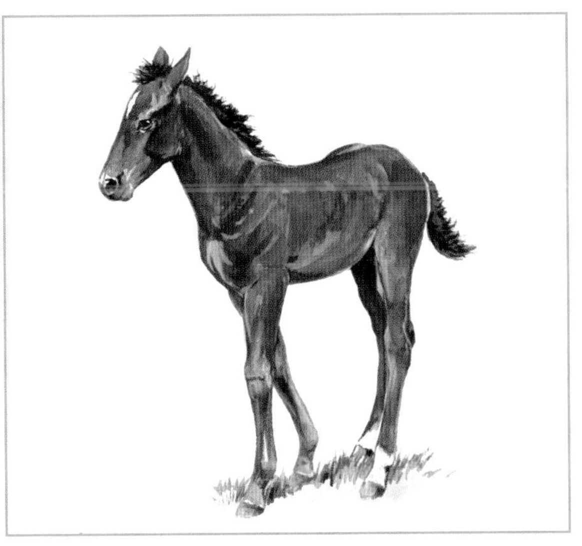

Sorrel. Ranges from coppery red to red. Mane and tail can be flaxen (golden), but are typically the same color as the body. There may be a dorsal stripe.

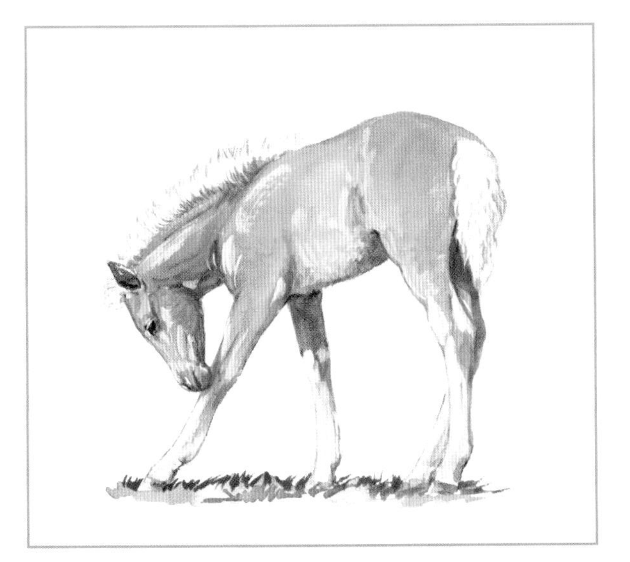

Palomino. Body color ranges from light to dark golden yellow. Mane and tail are white.

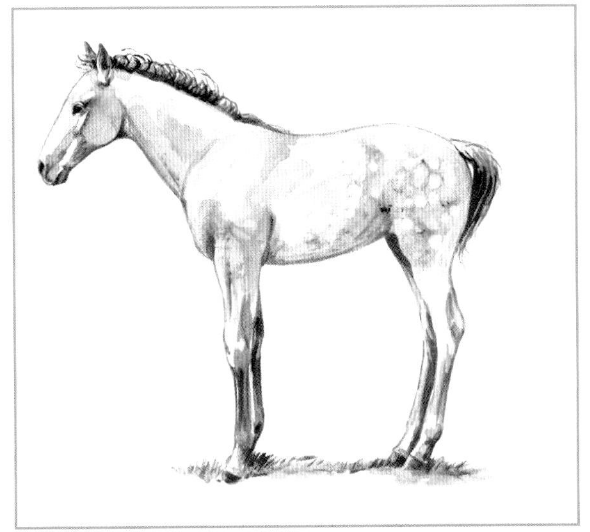

Gray. White hair is mixed with hair of other colors. Foals are often born solid or almost solid in color and then lighten with age. Dappling is common.

(continued on next page)

Common Horse Colors *(continued)*

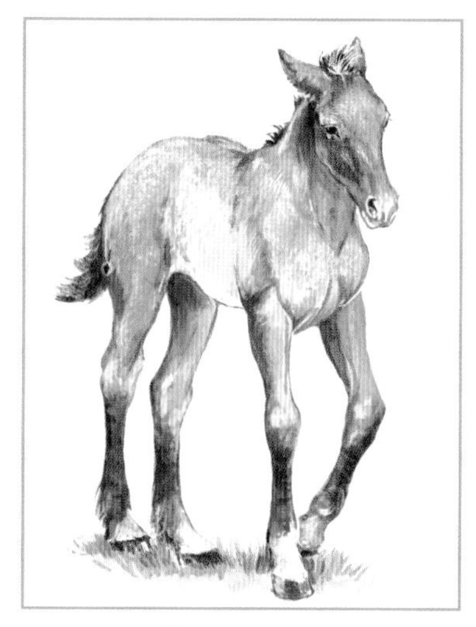

Roan. Can be chestnut, bay, brown, or black with white hairs running through the coat. Often difficult to distinguish from gray. There are blue roans and red roans, according to the combination of colors.

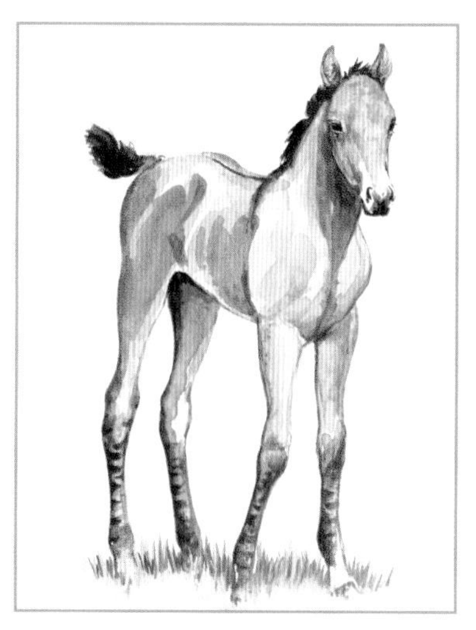

Dun. Body color is yellowish or golden; mane and tail are brown or black. There is a dorsal stripe. There may be black bars on the legs and a stripe across the withers.

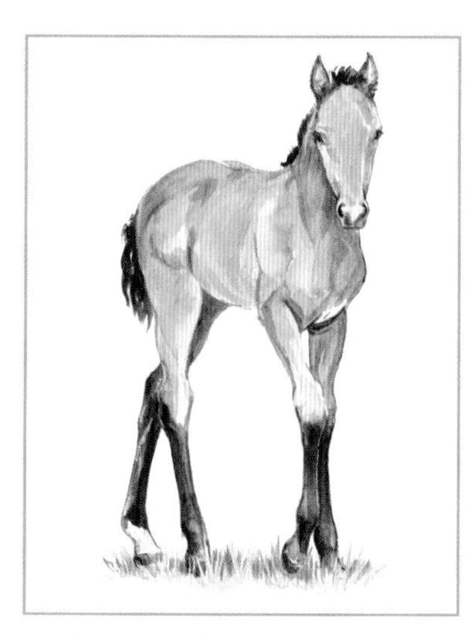

Buckskin. Yellow or golden body color with black mane and tail. Lower legs are black.

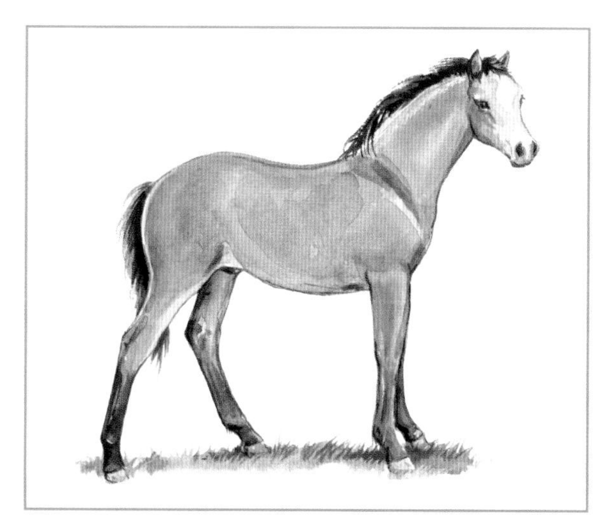

Grullo (also known as Grulla). Smoky or mouse-colored. Not a mixture of black and white hairs; instead, each hair is smoke- or mouse-colored. There are usually a dorsal stripe, shoulder striping or shadowing, and black bars on legs.

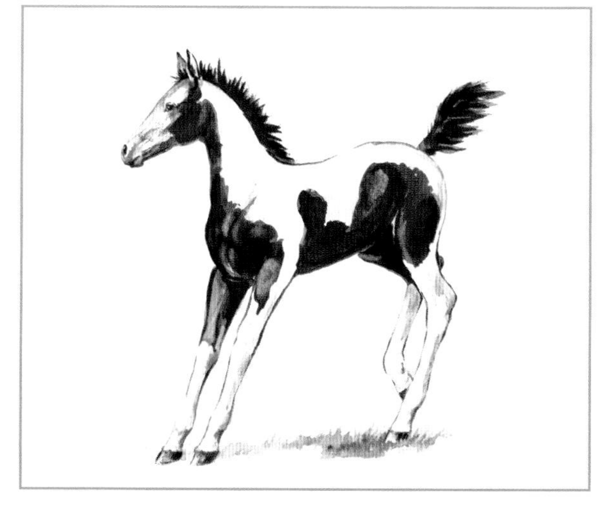

Pinto. White with colored patches. A black-and-white pinto is a **piebald;** nonblack-and-white is a **skewbald. Tobiano** is a white background with dark spots, while an **overo** is a dark horse with jagged patches of white.

Markings on the Face

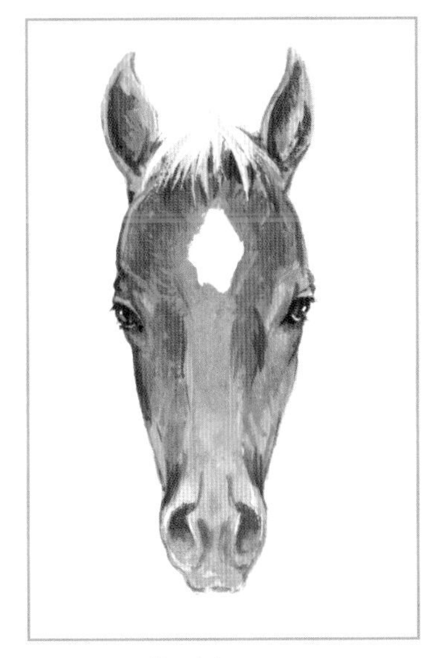

Star. Small white spot on forehead; can be diamond-shaped.

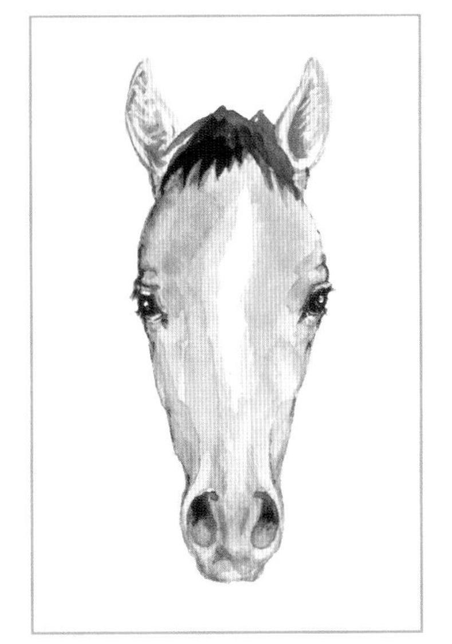

Strip. Very thin white marking down front of face; can be long or short.

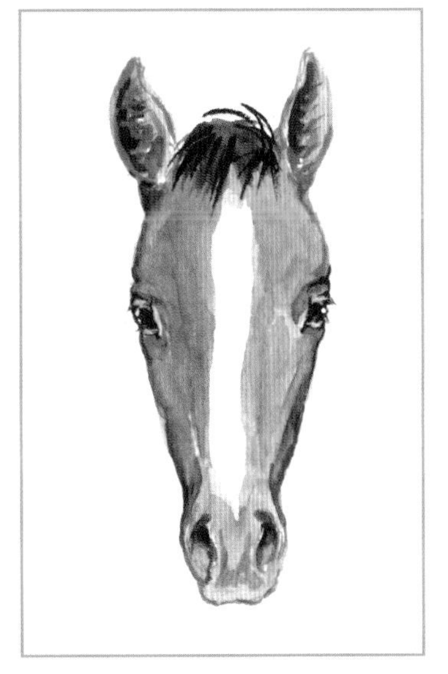

Blaze. Wide white marking between eyes and down front of face to muzzle, or including muzzle.

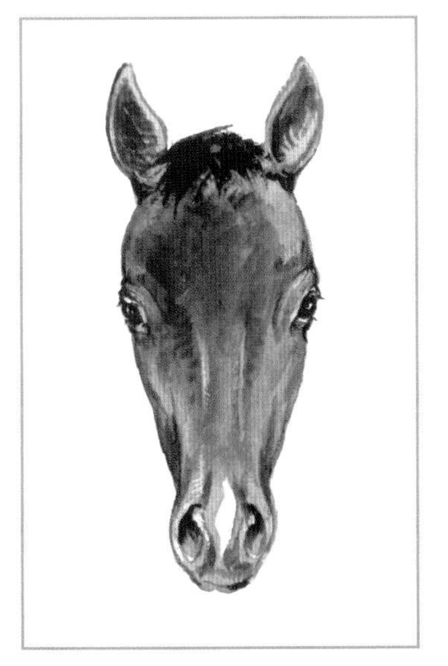

Snip. White or pink mark on muzzle between nostrils.

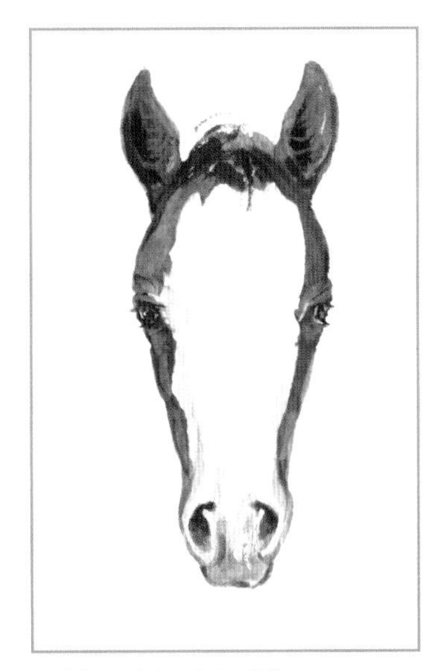

Bald. Bold white blaze covering much of face; may extend out around eyes or not.

Markings on the Legs

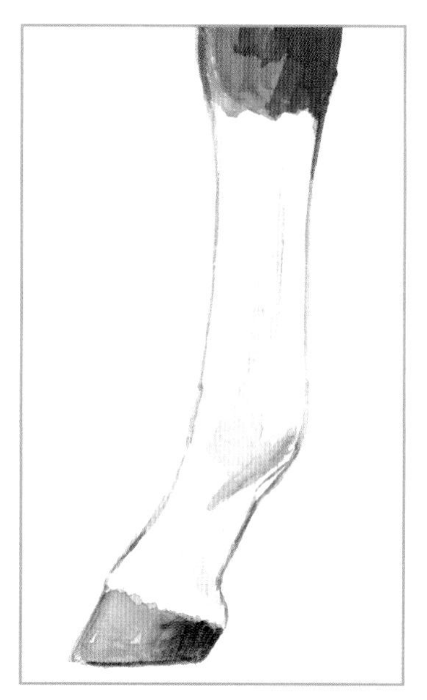

Stocking. White from just below knee or hock down to hoof.

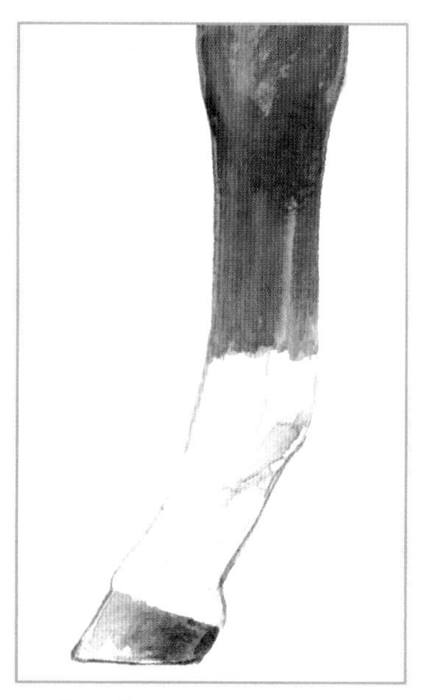

Sock. White runs about halfway from hoof to knee or hock.

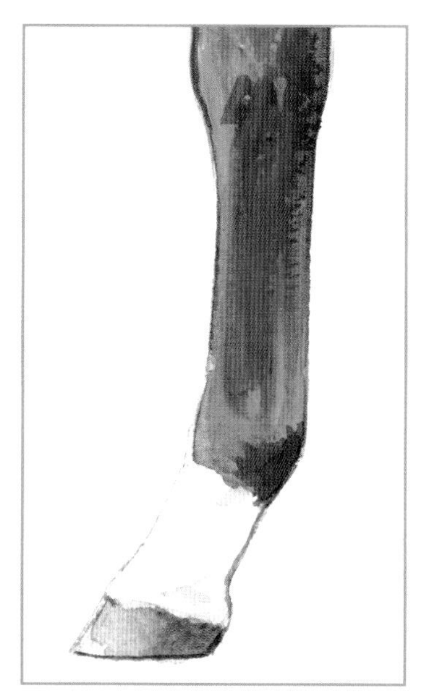

Pastern. Shorter than a sock; only the pastern area (above hoof, just below ankle) is white.

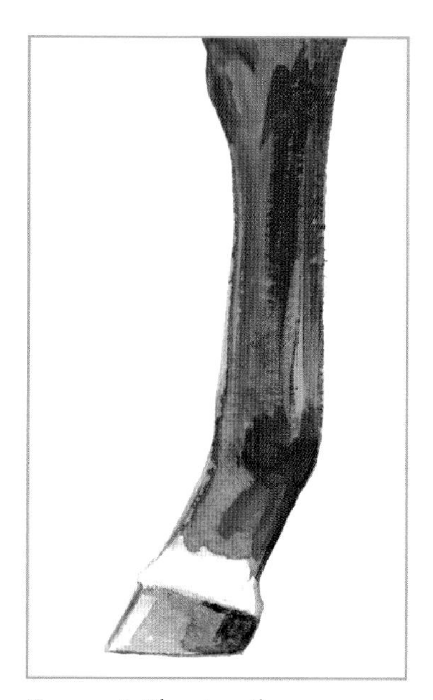

Coronet. Shorter than a pastern; just a small area right above the hoof is white.

Showing

Interested in showing? You don't have to wait until your horse can be ridden in order to compete. Most breed shows offer weanling halter classes, which are typically divided into fillies, colts, and geldings. These classes are open to weanlings of up to 1 year of age. (All weanlings are considered yearlings on January 1.) In these classes, weanlings are asked to walk, trot, and stand for the judge's inspection.

There are more choices for competition for yearlings, depending on your horse's breed and the particular show. As with weanlings, yearling halter classes are divided according to gender. There are also several different **in-hand classes** for yearlings, in which all horses are shown by the handler on the ground.

Happy Birthday!

Breed registries typically recognize January 1 as the horse's "official" birthday. In other words, the foal becomes a yearling on the first of January regardless of the actual date of his birth.

Yearling in-hand classes include Yearling Longe Line, in which yearlings are shown on a longe line at the walk, trot, and canter; they are also usually judged on conformation. Another good yearling class is the In-Hand Trail, which features obstacles similar to those found in a riding trail class.

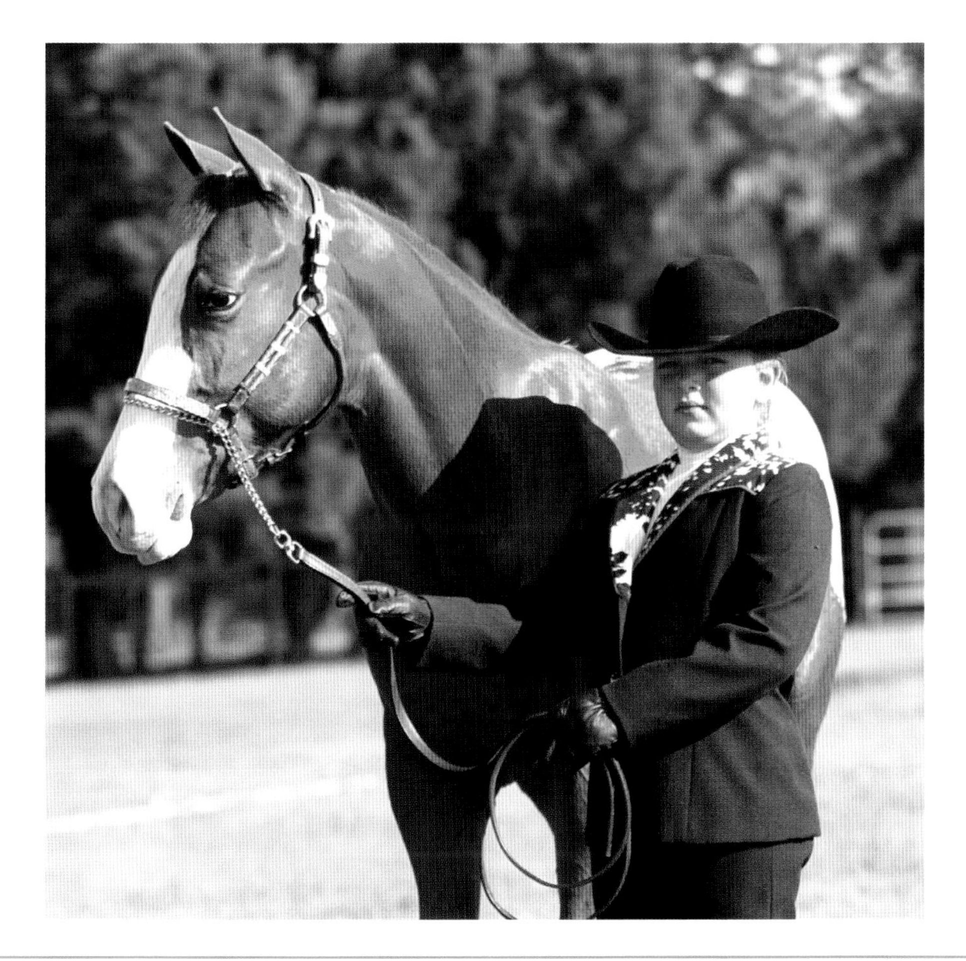

Weanling halter classes are a great way to expose a young horse to new experiences.

12

Record Keeping

Use this section to keep track of health care records and events you want to remember.

Veterinary Services Information

Veterinarian

Name: ______________________________

Address: ______________________________

____

____

Phone: ______________________________

Cell/pager: ______________________________

Backup veterinarian/clinic

Name: ______________________________

Address: ______________________________

____

____

Phone: ______________________________

Cell/pager: ______________________________

Other emergency contact

Name: ______________________________

Address: ______________________________

____

____

Phone: ______________________________

Cell/pager: ______________________________

Van transportation

Name: ______________________________

Address: ______________________________

____

____

Phone: ______________________________

Cell/pager: ______________________________

Breeding Information

MARE

Name: ______________________

Dates in heat: ______________________

Vet check

Date: ______________________

Comments: ______________________

Vet check

Date: ______________________

Comments: ______________________

Vet check

Date: ______________________

Comments: ______________________

Vet check

Date: ______________________

Comments: ______________________

Vet check

Date: ______________________

Comments: ______________________

Vet check

Date: ______________________

Comments: ______________________

Vet check

Date: ______________________

Comments: ______________________

STALLION

Name: ______________________

Stallion's farm

Name: ______________________

Address: ______________________

____

____

Phone: ______________________

Cell/pager: ______________________

Breeding dates

1st: ______________________

❑ A.I. (artificial insemination)

❑ live cover

2nd: ______________________

❑ A.I. ❑ live cover

Additional breeding dates: ______________________

❑ A.I. ❑ live cover

Comments: ______________________

____

____

DATE CHECKED IN-FOAL BY VETERINARIAN

Expected date of foaling: ______________________

Ultrasound

❑ Yes ❑ No

Comments: ______________________

____

Vet check

Date: ______________________

Comments: ______________________

Vet check

Date: ______________________

Comments: ______________________

Vet check

Date: ______________________

Comments: ______________________

Vet check

Date: ______________________

Comments: ______________________

Mare Vaccinations While Pregnant

The first semiannual vaccinations should be given during the fifth to sixth month of pregnancy. Follow up with booster shots four to six weeks prior to foaling due date. As a rule, veterinarians will give only killed (inactivated) agent vaccines to pregnant mares because a modified-live-virus vaccine must induce some type of infection to achieve immunization.

Equine encephalomyelitis

Dates: ______________________

Tetanus

Dates: ______________________

West Nile

Dates: ______________________

Influenza

Dates: ______________________

Rhinopneumonitis

Dates: ______________________

Other vaccinations

Kind: ______________________

Dates: ______________________

Kind: ______________________

Dates: ______________________

Kind: ______________________

Dates: ______________________

Kind: ______________________

Dates: ______________________

Kind: ______________________

Dates: ______________________

Deworming during Pregnancy

Date: ______________________

Type of dewormer: ______________________

Date: ______________________

Type of dewormer: ______________________

Date: ______________________

Type of dewormer: ______________________

Date: ______________________

Type of dewormer: ______________________

Date: ______________________

Type of dewormer: ______________________

Date: ______________________

Type of dewormer: ______________________

Date: ______________________

Type of dewormer: ______________________

Date: ______________________

Type of dewormer: ______________________

Date: ______________________

Type of dewormer: ______________________

Date: ______________________

Type of dewormer: ______________________

Date: ______________________

Type of dewormer: ______________________

Date: ______________________

Type of dewormer: ______________________

Mare's Feed

Feed

What kind: ______________________

Amount fed: ______________________

How many times daily: ______________________

Hay/pasture

What kind: ______________________

Amount fed: ______________________

How many times daily: ______________________

Changes in feed while pregnant

____

Comments: ______________________

Mare Hoof Care

Blacksmith

Name: ______________________

Address: ______________________

Phone: ______________________

Cell/pager: ______________________

Date

❑ Trimmed ❑ Shod

❑ New shoes ❑ Reset

Comments: ______________________

Date

❑ Trimmed ❑ Shod

❑ New shoes ❑ Reset

Comments: ______________________

Date

❑ Trimmed ❑ Shod

❑ New shoes ❑ Reset

Comments: ______________________

Date

❑ Trimmed ❑ Shod

❑ New shoes ❑ Reset

Comments: ______________________

Countdown to Foaling

Open Caslicks (if mare has one) 30 days before due date

Date opened: ____________________

Udder starting to fill out

Date first noticed: ____________________

Comments: ____________________

Muscles over croup and tail head start to soften

Date first noticed: ____________________

Mucus discharge/plug

Date passed: (typically passed within 72 hours of foaling) ____________________

Washed udder pre-foaling

Date done: ____________________

Edema (swelling) along lower belly

Date first noticed: ____________________

Wax on teats

Date and time first noticed: ____________

Leaking milk

Date and time first noticed: ____________

Comments: ____________________

____

____

____

____

____

Foaling Supplies Checklist

- ❑ Terry cloth towels (bath towel or half-size bath towels)
- ❑ Stainless-steel bucket
- ❑ Liquid soap such as Ivory, Dawn, or Joy
- ❑ Roll of cotton
- ❑ Baling twine or strong string
- ❑ Scissors
- ❑ Enemas (any enema safe for children is fine; a phosphate enema is best)
- ❑ Tincture of iodine* or Nolvasan solution for dipping navels
- ❑ Small plastic containers or 60 cc plastic syringe cases (for dipping foal's navel)
- ❑ Umbilical clamps or rubber bands (if foal's navel bleeds more than is normal)
- ❑ Obstetrical sleeves or plastic rectal sleeves
- ❑ Disposable tail wrap or gauze bandage (for wrapping tail)
- ❑ Disposable latex gloves
- ❑ Obstetric lubricant or K-Y Jelly
- ❑ Digital thermometer
- ❑ Small blanket or old down vest (in case you have to keep the foal warm on a cold night)
- ❑ Flashlights and batteries (in case of power failure)
- ❑ Cell phone or cordless phone
- ❑ Phone number of vets, experienced foaling person (keep list next to phone)

**Some vets use 2 percent iodine; others swear by the stronger 7 percent iodine. If you decide to use iodine to dip the navel, ask your vet which strength she recommends.*

Foaling Details

Water breaks

Date: ____________________

Time: ____________________

Comments: ____________________

Foal delivered

Time: ____________________

Sex: ____________________

Color: ____________________

Markings: ____________________

Approximate weight: ____________________

Name: ____________________

Nickname: ____________________

Comments: ____________________

Placenta passed

Time: ____________________

Comments: ____________________

Mare's udder washed postfoaling

Time: ____________________

Comments: ____________________

Foal stands

Time: ____________________

Comments: ____________________

Foal nurses first time

Time: ____________________

Comments: ____________________

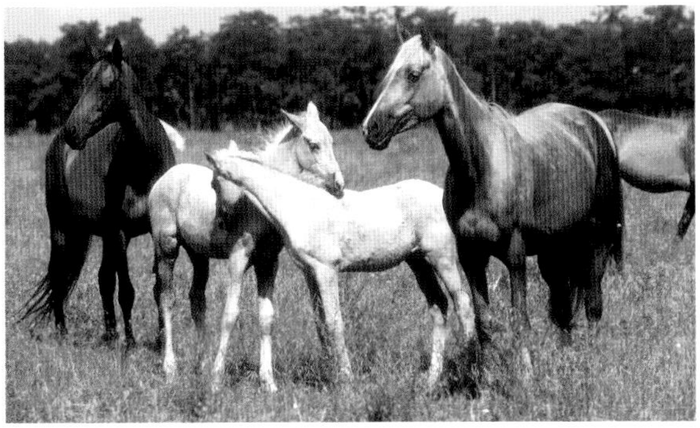

First 24 Hours Postfoaling

Bran mash(es) or wet feed for mare

When given: ______________________

Comments: ______________________

____

Deworm mare with ivermectin

When given: ______________________

Comments: ______________________

____

Enema given to foal

When given: ______________________

Comments: ______________________

____

Foal passes meconium

Time: ______________________

Comments: ______________________

____

Vet check for mare

Date: ______________________

Time: ______________________

Comments: ______________________

____

Vet check for foal (should be same day as mare's)

Date: ______________________

Time: ______________________

Comments: ______________________

____

BLOOD DRAWN FOR FOAL BLOOD TESTS

IgG test

Time: ______________________

Results and comments: ______________________

____

Complete blood count (CBC)

Time: ______________________

Results and comments: ______________________

____

Time spent outside day one

Where: ______________________

Home much time: ______________________

Comments: ______________________

____

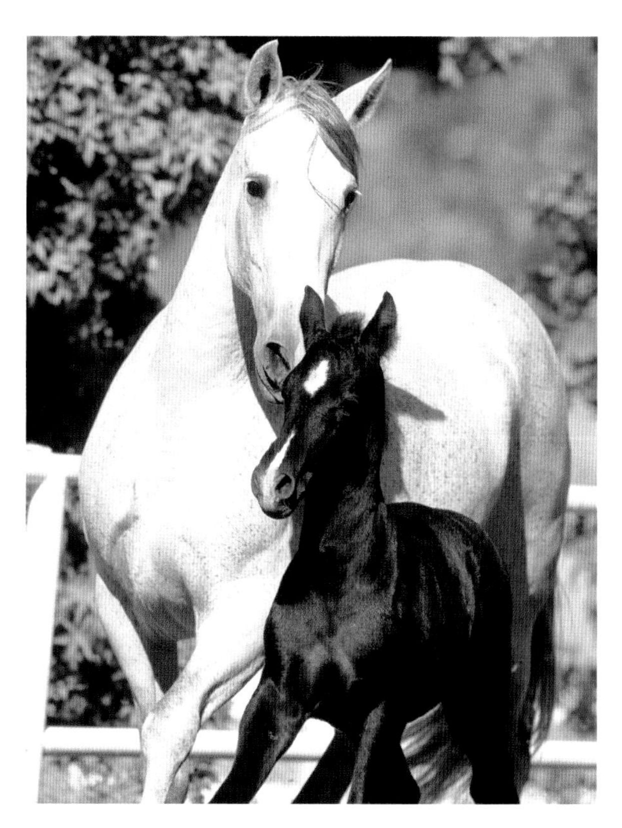

Welcome to the World!

Put your newborn foal's photo here.

Important Firsts

Learning to Lead

Date started: ____________________

Butt rope used: ❑ Yes ❑ No

Comments: ____________________

____

____

____

First Bath

Date: ____________________

Comments: ____________________

____

____

____

First Clipping

Date: ____________________

Comments: ____________________

____

____

____

Other Firsts

Date: ____________________

Comments: ____________________

____

____

____

Date: ____________________

Comments: ____________________

____

____

____

Other Firsts

Date: ____________________

Comments: ____________________

____

____

____

Date: ____________________

Comments: ____________________

____

____

____

Date: ____________________

Comments: ____________________

____

____

____

Date: ____________________

Comments: ____________________

____

____

____

MARE'S FOAL HEAT

First heat

Date: ____________________

Out of heat

Date: ____________________

Diarrhea in foal? ❑ Yes ❑ No

Treatment, if any: ____________________

Comments: ____________________

____

____

____

Blacksmith Visits and Hoof Care

Date

Trimmed: ______

Comments: ______

______

______

______

______

Date

Trimmed: ______

Comments: ______

______

______

______

______

Date

Trimmed: ______

Comments: ______

______

______

______

______

Date

Trimmed: ______

Comments: ______

______

______

______

______

Date

Trimmed: ______

Comments: ______

______

______

______

______

Foal's Feed

First noticed nibbling grain

Date: ______

First started eating grain/concentrate regularly

Date: ______

Kind: ______

Amount fed: ______

How many times daily: ______

Hay/pasture

What kind: ______

Amount fed: ______

How many times daily: ______

Changes in feed consumption

1 month: ______

2 months: ______

3 months: ______

4 months: ______

5 months: ______

6 months: ______

7 months: ______

8 months: ______

9 months: ______

10 months: ______

11 months: ______

12 months: ______

Foal Health

Temperature

Average: ____________________

General attitude

____

____

____

Comments: ____________________

____

____

____

WEANING

Weaned

Date: ____________________

Method used: ____________________

____

Comments: ____________________

____

____

____

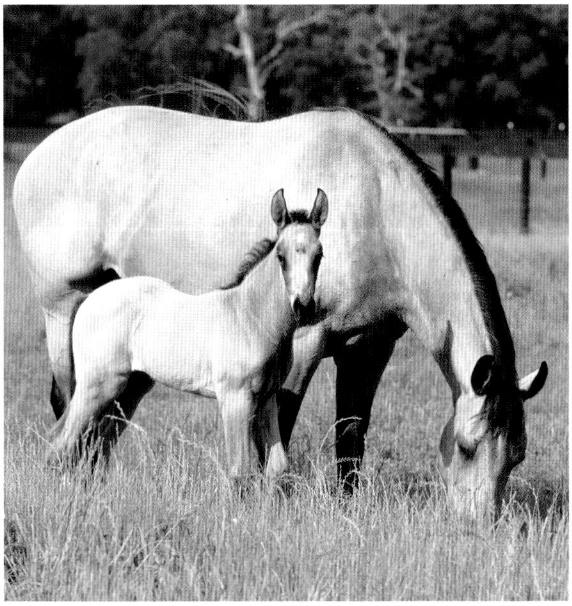

Vet Visits

Date: ____________________

Reason: ____________________

____

Comments: ____________________

____

____

____

Date: ____________________

Reason: ____________________

____

Comments: ____________________

____

____

____

Date: ____________________

Reason: ____________________

____

Comments: ____________________

____

____

____

Date: ____________________

Reason: ____________________

____

Comments: ____________________

____

____

____

Date: ____________________

Reason: ____________________

____

Comments: ____________________

____

____

____

Vaccinations

Equine encephalomyelitis

First dose: ______________________

Booster: ______________________

Booster: ______________________

Tetanus toxoid

First dose: ______________________

Booster: ______________________

Booster: ______________________

West Nile

First dose: ______________________

Booster: ______________________

Booster: ______________________

Influenza

First dose: ______________________

Booster: ______________________

Booster: ______________________

Rabies

First dose: ______________________

Booster: ______________________

Booster: ______________________

Other vaccinations

Kind: ______________________

Dates: ______________________

First dose: ______________________

Kind: ______________________

Dates: ______________________

First dose: ______________________

Kind: ______________________

Dates: ______________________

First dose: ______________________

Kind: ______________________

Dates: ______________________

First dose: ______________________

Foal Deworming

Date: ______________________

Type of dewormer: ______________________

Date: ______________________

Type of dewormer: ______________________

Date: ______________________

Type of dewormer: ______________________

Date: ______________________

Type of dewormer: ______________________

Date: ______________________

Type of dewormer: ______________________

Date: ______________________

Type of dewormer: ______________________

Date: ______________________

Type of dewormer: ______________________

Date: ______________________

Type of dewormer: ______________________

Date: ______________________

Type of dewormer: ______________________

Date: ______________________

Type of dewormer: ______________________

Date: ______________________

Type of dewormer: ______________________

Date: ______________________

Type of dewormer: ______________________

Glossary

Amniotic sac. Innermost membrane of the sac that enclosed the foal inside the placenta; also known as the amnion

Angular limb deformity. A limb that does not have correct conformation due to developmental problems in the joint angles

Antibodies. Proteins produced by the mare's body in response to contact with an antigen, which create immunity to the antigen when the foal absorbs these antibodies in her colostrum

Breech birth. The foal is backwards with his rump presented first. Immediate veterinary assistance is needed to save the foal.

Bridle path. Short, clipped area of the horse's mane directly behind the ears

Broodmare. Female horse used for breeding

Caslicks. A simple procedure done by a veterinarian to sew the vulva lips partially closed to prevent infection in the mare; must be cut open before foaling

Colostrum. The first fluid produced by the mammary glands, rich in protein and protective antibodies

Colt. Ungelded male horse 4 years old and younger

Concentrate. Any type of grain or pelleted feed used to supplement the horse's forage

Conformation. A horse's physical build and bodily proportions

Congenital. A condition present at birth.

Coprophagia. The behavior of eating manure. Common in young foals.

Coronary band. Area where the hair meets the hoof. Also known as the coronet.

Cryptorchid. Male horse of any age with one or both testicles not descended; usually requires abdominal surgery for castration

Dam. Female parent of a horse

"Dummy" foal. Brain swelling develops within first 24 hours due to lack of oxygen during birthing process

Embryo. Unborn foal in the early stages of development up to the third month of gestation

Epiphysitis. Inflammation in the growth plates at the ends of the long bones, such as the cannon bone. Affected areas may show swelling, tenderness, and heat.

Equine encephalomyelitis. Viral disease spread by mosquitoes; also known as "sleeping sickness"

Farrier. Blacksmith, horseshoer

Fetus. Unborn foal, after the third month of gestation

Filly. Female horse 4 years old and younger

Foal. Young horse of either sex; also the act of giving birth

Foal heat. The mare's first heat, which occurs 6 to 12 days after foaling.

Forage. Roughage consisting of pasture and/or hay; forage should make up the bulk of the horse's diet

Gelding. Male horse of any age that has been castrated (had both testicles removed); also the act of castration

Gestation. Pregnancy

Hippomanes. Small, free-floating rubbery mass of tissue found in the placenta

IgG test. Blood test used to determine if newborn foal has received enough antibodies from his dam's colostrum; also known as failure of passive transfer test

Influenza. Upper respiratory disease caused by virus

Jaundiced-foal syndrome. Occurs when the foal's blood type is incompatible with his dam's. In this case, antibodies in the mare's colostrum actually fight against the foal's red blood cells. Foal must be bottle-fed and not be allowed to nurse until testing shows the absence of these antibodies.

Lactation. Period of time the broodmare is nursing her foal

Maiden. Female horse that has never had a foal; can also refer to a female that has never been bred

Mare. Female horse age 5 and older

Mastitis. Inflammation of the udder

Meconium. First bowel movement of the newborn foal

Neonatal maladjustment syndrome. Can result from brain damage due to trauma during birth. Affected foal may exhibit seizures, convulsions, and other neurological signs.

Passive immunity. Protection from antibodies passed to foal through the mare's colostrum

Placenta. Organ that develops within the uterus to carry the fetus until birth

Plasma. Unclotted blood with red cells removed

Presentation. Position of the foal in the birth canal at delivery

Red-bag foaling. Situation when part of placenta comes through the birth canal ahead of the foal; caused by placenta detaching from the uterus too soon

Rhinopneumonitis. Can cause abortion in pregnant mares, respiratory disease, and nervous system disorders; mares should be vaccinated for it during gestation

Rotavirus A. Virus that causes diarrhea in foals; mares should be vaccinated for it in late gestation

Sclera. White part of the eye

Scours. Diarrhea, loose stool

Septicemia. Infection of the bloodstream

Sire. Male parent of a horse

Stallion. Male horse used for breeding

Strangles. Bacterial respiratory disease

Suckling. Nursing foal of any age up until weaning

Tetanus, Lockjaw. Infection caused by bacteria that can occur when a wound is infected

Umbilical cord. Cord attached to the unborn foal at the navel that connects it to the placenta so that the foal receives oxygen and nourishment before birth

Uterine prolapse. The expelling of the entire uterus after foaling; must be treated immediately in order to save the mare

Uterus. Hollow organ inside the mare in which the foal contained in the placenta develops during pregnancy

Weanling. Foal less than 1 year old that has been separated from his mother and is no longer nursing

West Nile virus. Encephalitis virus spread by mosquitoes to birds, horses, humans

Yearling. Young horse of either sex in its second year of life after January 1, when it is considered 1 year old

Breed Associations

American Hanoverian Society, Inc.
4067 Iron Works Parkway, Suite 1
Lexington, KY 40511
859-255-4141
www.hanoverian.org

American Holsteiner Horse Association
222 East Main Street, #1
Georgetown, KY 40324
502-863-4239
www.holsteiner.com

American Miniature Horse Association, Inc.
5601 South Interstate 35 W
Alvarado, TX 76009
817-783-5600
www.amha.com

American Morgan Horse Association, Inc.
P. O. Box 960
Shelburne, VT 05482
802-985-4944
www.morganhorse.com

American Paint Horse Association
P. O. Box 961023
Fort Worth, TX 76161
817-834-2742
www.apha.com

American Quarter Horse Association
P. O. Box 200
Amarillo, TX 79168
806-376-4811
www.aqha.com

American Saddlebred Horse Association
4093 Iron Works Parkway
Lexington, KY 40511
859-259-2742
www.saddlebred.com

American Shetland Pony Club
81-B E. Queenwood
Morton, IL 61550
309-263-4044
www.shetlandminiature.com

American Trakehner Association, Inc.
1514 West Church Street
Newark, OH 43055
740-344-1111
www.americantrakehner.com

American Warmblood Society
2 Buffalo Run Road
Center Ridge, AR 72027
501-893-2777
www.americanwarmblood.org

Appaloosa Horse Club, Inc.
2720 West Pullman Road
Moscow, ID 83843
208-882-5578
www.appaloosa.com

Arabian Horse Registry of America, Inc.
10805 East Bethany Drive
Aurora, CO 80014
303-696-4500
www.theregistry.org

Gypsy Vanner Horse Society
P. O. Box 772407
Ocala, FL 34477
352-347-9573
www.gypsyvannerhorse.com

International Buckskin Horse Association
P. O. Box 268
Shelby, IN 46377
219-552-1013
www.ibha.net

Missouri Fox Trotting Horse Breed Association, Inc.
P. O. Box 1027
Ava, MO 65608
417-683-2468
www.mfthba.com

National Show Horse Registry
10368 Bluegrass Parkway
Louisville, KY 40299
502-266-5100
www.nshregistry.org

National Spotted Saddle Horse Association
P. O. Box 898
Murfreesboro, TN 37133
615-890-2864
www.nssha.com

Palomino Horse Breeders of America
15253 East Skelly Drive
Tulsa, OK 74116
918-438-1234
www.palominohba.com

Paso Fino Horse Association, Inc.
101 North Collins Street
Plant City, FL 33563
813-719-7777
www.pfha.org

Peruvian Paso Horse Registry of North America
3077 Wiljan Court, Suite A
Santa Rosa, CA 95407
707-579-4394
www.pphrna.org

Pinto Horse Association of America, Inc.
7330 North West 23rd Street
Bethany, OK 73008
405-491-0111
www.pinto.org

Pony of the Americas Club, Inc.
5240 Elmwood Avenue
Indianapolis, IN 46203
317-788-0107
www.poac.org

Rocky Mountain Horse Association
P. O. Box 129
Mt. Olivet, KY 41064
606-724-2354
www.rmhorse.com

Spanish Mustang Registry, Inc.
11790 Halstad Avenue
Lonsdale, MN 55046
507-744-2704
www.spanishmustang.org

Tennessee Walking Horse Breeders' and Exhibitors' Association
P. O. Box 286
Lewisburg, TN 37091
931-359-1574
www.twhbea.com

The Jockey Club (Thoroughbreds)
821 Corporate Drive
Lexington, KY 40503
859-224-2700
www.jockeyclub.com

United States Trotting Association (Standardbreds)
750 Michigan Avenue
Columbus, OH 43215
614-224-2291
www.ustrotting.com

Welsh Pony and Cob Society of America, Inc.
P. O. Box 2977
Winchester, VA 22604
540-667-6195
www.welshpony.org

Clubs & Organizations

American Association of Equine Practitioners
4075 Iron Works Parkway
Lexington, KY 40511
859-233-0147
www.aaep.org

American Driving Society
2324 Clark Road
Lapeer, MI 48446
810-664-8666
www.americandrivingsociety.org

American Horse Council
1616 H Street North West, 7th Floor
Washington, DC 20006
202-296-4031
www.horsecouncil.org

Intercollegiate Horse Show Association
P. O. Box 741
Stony Brook, NY 11790
631-751-2803
www.ihsa.com

National Cutting Horse Association
260 Bailey Avenue
Fort Worth, TX 76107
817-244-6188
www.nchacutting.com

National FFA Organization
P. O. Box 68960
Indianapolis, IN 46268
317-802-6060
www.ffa.org

National 4-H Council
www.4husa.org
Type in your state for detailed information about 4-H in your area.

National Reining Horse Association
3000 North West 10th Street
Oklahoma City, OK 73107
405-946-7400
www.nrha.com

North American Riding for the Handicapped Association
P. O. Box 33150
Denver, CO 80233
303-452-1212
www.narha.org

United States Dressage Federation
220 Lexington Green Circle, Suite 510
Lexington, KY 40503
859-971-2277
www.usdf.org

United States Equestrian Team
Pottersville Road
Gladstone, NJ 07934
908-234-1251
www.uset.org

United States Pony Clubs, Inc.
4041 Iron Works Parkway
Lexington, KY 40511
859-254-7669
www.ponyclub.org

Foaling Alarm Systems

Birth Alarm has a transmitter attached to a leather girth that is placed around the mare's withers. The girth isn't uncomfortable for the mare, but when she lies down totally flat on her side, as is customary in foaling, the transmitter activates the alarm after a few seconds. The transmitter's range can be extended by attaching it to a pager. (This type of alarm system is also used to summon help for horses prone to colic.)
Birth Alarm
800-581-8666
www.birthalarmusa.com

Breeder Alert utilizes a small radio transmitter encased in a leather pouch that is attached to the mare's halter. Once the mare lies flat out, as most do when foaling, the transmitter sends a signal through the receiver, which signals a pager. There is a built-in delay of ten seconds if the mare should lie down and then get up. (This system is also helpful should a horse get cast in his stall or lie down because of colic.)
Breeder Alert
www.breederalert.com

Foal-ALERT is a system that requires a small transmitter be sutured to the mare's vulva by your veterinarian. The system is activated when the vulva lips physically open, typically by the foal's foot or sometimes by the mare straining in labor. Once the transmitter is activated, the receiver sounds an audible alarm and any attached accessories, such as pagers, are also activated.
Foal-ALERT
800-237-8861
www.foalert.com

Books

Gower, Jeanette. *Horse Color Explained: A Breeder's Perspective.* Trafalgar Square, 1999.
A helpful guide that explains the principles behind horse coat color and markings.

Web sites

www.4aHORSE.com
www.lynnpalm.com
www.parelli.com
www.ttouch.com (Linda Tellington-Jones: TTouch Equine Awareness Method and Tellington TTouch Training)

For more information about horse colors:

http://members.aol.com/battyatty/
www.champagnehorses.org
www.doubledilute.com
www.equinecolor.com
www.horsecolor.com

Index

Other Storey Titles You Will Enjoy

The Horse Behavior Problem Solver, by Jessica Jahiel. Using a friendly question-and-answer format and drawing on real-life case studies, Jahiel explains how a horse thinks and learns, why it acts the way it does, and how you should respond. 352 pages. Paperback. ISBN 1-58017-524-4.

Horse Care for Kids, by Cherry Hill. For kids who are eager to learn the essentials of equine care, Hill teaches everything they need to know to become a responsible and successful horse or pony owner. 128 pages. Paperback. ISBN 1-58017-407-8.

The Horse Conformation Handbook, by Heather Smith Thomas. Horse conformation-how the shape and form of a particular horse's body compares to an anatomical ideal-affects a horse's performance and suitability for particular functions. This detailed "tour of the horse" analyzes all aspects of conformation that are critical for every horse owner to understand. 400 pages. Paperback. ISBN 1-58017-558-9.

The Horse Doctor Is In, by Brent Kelley, DVM. Drawing from his decades of experience, veterinarian Brent Kelley shares practical information on all the topics of concern to horse owners—including disease prevention and treatment, lameness, breeding and foaling, and general horse care and management—through real-life stories about horses, owners, trainers, and breeders. 416 pages. Paperback. ISBN 1-58017-460-4.

Storey's Guide to Raising Horses, by Heather Smith Thomas. Whether you are an experienced horse handler or are planning to own your first horse, this complete guide to intelligent horsekeeping covers all aspects of keeping a horse fit and healthy in body and spirit. 512 pages. Paperback. ISBN 1-58017-127-3.

Storey's Guide to Training Horses, by Heather Smith Thomas. This comprehensive guide covers every aspect of the training process-from basic safety to retraining a horse that has developed a bad habit-this is an essential handbook for all horse owners. 512 pages. Paperback. ISBN 1-58017-467-1.

Storey's Horse-Lover's Encyclopedia, edited by Deborah Burns. This comprehensive, user-friendly, A-to-Z guide to all things equine covers breeds, tack, facilities, daily care, health issues, riding styles, shows, and much more. 480 pages. Paperback. ISBN 1-58017-317-9.

Metric Conversion Chart

Use this chart to convert the U.S. measurements in this book to metric.

If you have:	Multiply by:	To find:
inches	x 25	= millimeters
feet	x 30	= centimeters
ounces	x 28	= grams
pounds	x 0.45	= kilograms
fluid ounces	x 30	= milliliters
pints, U.S.	x 0.47	= liters
quarts, U.S.	x 0.95	= liters
gallons, U.S.	x 3.8	= liters